AMERICANS
AT MIDLIFE

AMERICANS AT MIDLIFE

Caught between Generations

Rosalie G. Genovese

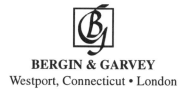

BERGIN & GARVEY
Westport, Connecticut • London

Library of Congress Cataloging-in-Publication Data

Genovese, Rosalie G.
   Americans at midlife : caught between generations / Rosalie G.
Genovese.
      p. cm.
   Includes bibliographical references and index.
   ISBN 0-89789-466-9 (alk. paper)
   1. Middle aged persons—United States—Life skills guides.
   I. Title.
   HQ1059.5.U5G46   1997
   305.24′4—DC20   96-41448

British Library Cataloguing in Publication Data is available.

Library of Congress Catalog Card Number: 96-41448
ISBN: 0-89789-466-9

First published in 1997

Bergin & Garvey, 88 Post Road West, Westport, CT 06881
An imprint of Greenwood Publishing Group, Inc.

Printed in the United States of America

The paper used in this book complies with the
Permanent Paper Standard issued by the National
Information Standards Organization (Z39.48–1984).

10 9 8 7 6 5 4 3 2 1

For Frank

Contents

Preface

For some years, I have been studying the impact of public policies on individuals and families. A particular research interest has been an analysis of how groups develop informal solutions in the absence of organized programs to meet needs, in areas such as education, social programs or help with disabled family members. Groups also arise for individuals and families with special needs and provide them with information, services and support.

More recently, the challenges and responsibilities of midlife have become a focus of interest as friends, colleagues and acquaintances respond to changes in family composition and relationships. The issues of midlife include such things as young adults not leaving home as readily as their parents at their age, or the impact of divorce, nontraditional relationships or unemployment on family members. Above all, the almost universal preoccupation with aging parents is the issue that led me to write this book. Those of us fortunate enough at midlife to have living parents wonder about how they will spend their last years and whether they will continue to be independent or need care.

These concerns lead many individuals to realize that their vision of midlife as a time for relaxation and enjoyment often can be inaccurate. Some mid-life Americans are concerned about their current and future economic security. Regardless of whether their incomes are large or small, Americans at midlife are planning for the longer lives they hope to have. At the same time, those at midlife today have many advantages as longer life expectancy offers opportunities for continued or new chances to change and develop new interests, experiences and relationships.

In writing this book, I searched through many sources of information on how to make these mid-life tasks easier. Resources on financial planning, relationships with adult children and aging parents and related topics have been put together in one place. The material in the book will direct readers toward information about a topic of interest. They also are advised to consult experts in specific fields for in-depth assistance, especially concerning financial and legal matters. Regulations and laws change frequently, and more up-to-date facts may be available.

My thanks go to those friends and colleagues who contributed suggestions and information. I especially want to thank my good friend and colleague, Sylvia F. Fava, who is always ready to listen, discuss questions and generously offer her expert opinion, no matter how busy she is. Bryna Rubinger, long-time friend, provided valuable insights from her work as a gerontology professional. Special thanks also go to Nan Johnson, Director of the Susan B. Anthony University Center at the University of Rochester, where I was a visiting scholar while writing this book.

As always, I owe a debt to Frank who has encouraged me and endured my idiosyncrasies and preoccupation during the preparation of this manuscript. He also provided technical assistance when I struggled with a new computer and software program, both seemingly determined to thwart me at the most inopportune times. This book is dedicated to him, in recognition of the midlife issues and experiences we have shared.

Abbreviations

AARP	American Association of Retired Persons
CAPS	Children of Aging Parents
CBO	Congressional Budget Office
CDF	Children's Defense Fund
DCAP	Dependent Care Assistance Program
DOL	Department of Labor
EEOC	Equal Employment Opportunity Commission
EITC or EIC	Earned Income Credit
ERISA	Employee Retirement Income Security Act
GAP	Grandparents as Parents
HHS	U.S. Department of Health and Human Services
IRA	Individual Retirement Account
IRS	Internal Revenue Service
IWPR	Institute for Women's Policy Research
NSCLC	National Senior Citizens Law Center
NSFH	National Survey of Families and Households
OWL	Older Women's League
QDRO	Qualified Domestic Relations Court Order
ROCKING	Raising Our Children's Kids: An Intergenerational Network of Grandparenting
SCORE	Service Corps of Retired Executives
SEP	Simplified Employee Pension
SSA	Social Security Administration
SSI	Supplemental Security Income

CHAPTER 1

Midlife: An Introduction

The meaning of midlife is changing for individuals and families. Social scientists also are reassessing how it fits into the life course of individuals and families. Defining midlife as the "empty nest" period of life is inaccurate for many Americans whose children still live at home; for many, childbearing and childrearing responsibilities have not ended by midlife. Some have both children who are toddlers and others who are finishing college. Some are even grandparents who unexpectedly find themselves raising grandchildren.

Longer life-expectancy also influences our changing perspectives on midlife. Adults in their 50s who are making wide-ranging plans for the future may contemplate a new career or remarriage; retirement may be thought of as a distant event. Their later life patterns may differ from those of many current retirees who left the work force while they were still in their 50s, often as a result of employers' attractive early retirement offers.

EFFECTS OF DEMOGRAPHIC AND SOCIAL CHANGES ON MIDLIFE

The changing demographics of the American population are affecting how midlife is viewed. The period is being transformed into a time of challenges and complex decisions as Americans are living longer. Changes in marital status, family composition and intergenerational relationships affect Americans at midlife and beyond. Moreover, increased longevity is a crucial factor in their planning for the future.

Demographic and social changes affecting mid-life Americans include a tendency to marry later than their parents did. In fact, their age at marriage is similar to the ages of young people at the turn of the century. The average age at marriage in 1990 was 26 years for men and 24 years for women (Shapiro 1991). But Americans do not necessarily stay married. Divorce rates have increased dramatically, with almost one marriage in two ending in divorce. Baby-boom women, now between the ages of 30 and 44, are the most likely group in American history to divorce during their lifetimes (Norton and Miller 1992).

As we know, however, Americans have not given up on marriage. They tend to remarry and create blended families. Such families may consist of children from previous marriages and the current marriage; sometimes "his," "hers" and "theirs." According to the Census Bureau, 4 out of 10 marriages represent a second marriage for one or both partners.

Childrearing may extend farther into midlife as many women have children when they are older. An estimated 20 percent of first births are to mothers over 30 years of age (Shapiro 1991). Moreover, new technology and practices like in-vitro fertilization and surrogate mothers have blurred the meaning of menopause as the end of childbearing for women. Women who remarry often have children, but even some mid-life couples are choosing to have an additional child after their others are grown.

The traditional family of father in the work force and mother at home with the children represents a small proportion of all families. With increased divorce and single-parent families, more children spend part of their childhood in single parent and step families. More than 50 percent of black children live with a single parent, compared to 19 percent of white and 30 percent of Hispanic children. In 1988, 4.7 million children lived with a never-married parent, and an additional 5.9 million lived with a divorced parent (Saluter 1989, 5).

With the trend toward women entering and remaining in the labor force after marriage, the two-income family has become common. Dual-earner couples and single-parent families are dominant family types in the United States (O'Rand, Henretta, and Krecker 1992, 81). Today, two incomes have become essential to many families' economic security, whether to achieve incomes above the poverty level or to maintain a middle-income lifestyle.

More Americans are single today than twenty years ago for a variety of reasons, including postponed marriages and high divorce rates (Saluter 1989, 1). Older Americans, often women, are remaining single after the death of a spouse. Given the differences in the life-expectancy of women and men, many women will outlive their spouses and are less likely than men to remarry.

Some women and men will never marry. The proportion of never-married is higher for African Americans than for whites. For example, three-quarters of African-American women had not been married by their early 20s in 1988, compared to 59 percent of white women (Saluter 1989, 2). A higher proportion of Hispanics than whites also had never been married.

Other trends affecting mid-life families are the aging of the population and increased longevity. There was a 22 percent increase in the population over 65 during the 1980s. The number of Americans over 80, about 6.9 million in 1990, could reach 29 million by the year 2050 (Taeuber 1992, v). This trend means that Americans will spend more years in retirement, with important implications for financial planning and economic security. The impact of these changes on individuals and families is analyzed throughout this book.

WHAT IS MIDLIFE?

Such demographic and social changes help explain why images of, and attitudes toward, midlife are changing. Midlife is a period without clear boundaries and can be defined roughly as the years from 40 to 60. However, some analysts would have midlife start at 35 years; for others, it ends at 65 or even 69 years (Troll 1989; Bumpass and Aquilino 1995; Zal 1992). For Troll, midlife begins when the children are grown. Brubaker (1985, 14) would not even define midlife by chronological age, since individuals marry and have children at different ages. Some individuals have several families, as when older men with grown children marry younger women and become parents again. According to Zal, over 50 million Americans, or one-quarter of the population, is considered middle-aged. These numbers will increase with baby boomers who turned 50 in 1996.

Regardless of its boundaries, social scientists tend to focus on two major aspects of midlife: the "empty nest," after the children have left home, and retirement. Psychologists often considered this period a traumatic time for women who might be depressed about the end of childrearing and the launching of their children. They might be unsure of what to do with the rest of their lives (see Sheehy 1977). Friedan (1993) has a much more optimistic perspective on mid- and later life, as is evident in her book's title, *The Fountain of Age*. Despite these differing perspectives on the implications of the empty nest, this phase is coming later for many families as adult children continue to live at home. In general, smaller families and longer life spans mean fewer years spent raising children (Brubaker 1985, 17). For those who marry several times, however, this phase may be lengthened with the existence of several families.

In the adult development literature of the 1960s and 1970s, midlife seemed to mark the end of growth, to be followed by retirement, old age and gradual decline (see, for example, Levinson 1978). To Cumming and Henry (1961), mid-life adults began the process of "disengagement" from society, a winding down of social activity.

With Americans living longer and more actively well into their 70s, 80s or beyond, this view of midlife does not fit the reality. They are not ready to contemplate "being put out to pasture." Women may be relieved, not depressed, to see their children launched. This milestone allows many to concentrate wholeheartedly on their careers, not retirement. Mid-life men and women who are at the peak of their careers want to continue to be productive. For some, this time of life may mean concentrating on new interests or new careers. In *The Fountain of Age*, Betty Friedan (1993) takes the adult development movement to task for considering midlife almost as an ending, with little growth still to occur.

Recent interest in midlife among researchers and practitioners gave rise to the Network on Successful Midlife Development (MIDMAC), funded by the John D. and Catherine T. MacArthur Foundation's program in Health and Human Development. Network members in the social sciences and medicine have undertaken wide-ranging studies of midlife. Their view of midlife as an active part of the life course is evident from their use of "successful" in their title, as well as in their research topics and findings (see, for example, Bumpass and Aquilino 1995).

In recent years, midlife often has been pictured as "the good years," a time for relaxing and enjoying leisure time after the children are grown. Advertisements for exotic vacations or second homes show active, vigorous and well-to-do couples in their middle years with the time and resources to do what they want. Mid-life women and men often are shown beginning new careers or pursuing avocations, often because their affluence allows them to take risks.

But alongside these rosy vignettes are unsettling pictures of other Americans at midlife. The demographic and structural changes discussed earlier affect families' well-being in midlife and retirement. Economic security is an unattainable goal for many individuals and families whose lives are a constant struggle for survival. For example, consider a single mother simultaneously raising her own and her young daughter's children. Her full "nest" and extended childrearing years add to her economic and social responsibilities. She may have to postpone her long-awaited retirement to meet the needs of this extended family.

Other women, alone at midlife, may approach their later years with few resources as a result of minimum-wage jobs, divorce or widowhood. Some have worked at low-paying jobs all of their lives, without health and retirement benefits or the ability to save for retirement.

Mid-life men also may be insecure financially as a result of low-paying skills, plant closings or corporate layoffs. Black males especially have suffered from the decline in blue-collar jobs offering good pay and benefits as corporations have sought cheaper labor in other countries. Even many two-income families have not achieved the economic security they had expected.

Other mid-life responsibilities create stress and uncertainty for the well-to-do as well as for those with low incomes. At the turn of the century, few parents lived until their children reached midlife. Today's mid-life adults may expect their parents to live until their 80s or 90s and to need care. Some mid-life families face simultaneous care responsibilities for older *and* younger generations. The term "sandwich generation" describes the strains experienced by such couples. Women not in the labor force have traditionally cared for aging parents, but the majority of women work today. Providing or arranging elder care is a major added responsibility for them (Shapiro 1991, 5). It is a big addition to their already tight schedules.

Despite the attention given to the pressures on the sandwich generation, studies (Taeuber 1992; Loomis and Booth 1995; Bumpass and Aquilino1995) have indicated that the number of families whose parents need care while their children are still at home is relatively small. Families in this situation, however, may be weighed down by the conflicting demands on their time and financial resources. Also, with delayed childbearing, more women in the future will be trying to raise children and care for parents at the same time. A colleague of mine heard mid-life adults described as part of a club sandwich, with the layers made up of four generations--their aging parents, themselves, their young adult children and grandchildren.

Families are "squeezed" by other responsibilities as well. A woman may be caring simultaneously for an ailing husband and an aging parent. Other families are pressured economically when they try to save for their children's education, a secure retirement, and financially assist their parents when necessary. A job loss for one or both partners is devastating both economically and psychologically.

Given the uncertainty surrounding employment and a lengthening retirement period, planning for the present and the future has become more important than ever at midlife. Since people are living longer, they can expect to spend more time in retirement, start second careers, or make major career changes.

The diversity of circumstances and patterns at midlife will be highlighted throughout this book. Some families, free of financial and caregiving worries, look forward to living as well in retirement as they do now; for others, the future presents many worries, while those in between are managing adequately and expect to continue to do so. Ethnic and cultural differences in family composition and lifestyles also are identified in the chapters that follow.

An important issue for mid-life Americans is the government's role in ensuring the economic well-being of its citizens. We are seeing a shift away from government's acceptance of responsibility to provide a safety net for those in need--especially children and the elderly--toward an emphasis on self-reliance. Efforts to shrink government's role in health care and other entitlements jeopardize the well-being of the elderly, as do politicians' speeches praising individual responsibility and informal, volunteer community supports. Cuts in government programs will make it more difficult for low-income families to move out of poverty, achieve economic stability and prepare for their later years. The decreasing proportion of older Americans classified as poor may be reversed by program cuts implemented to meet the goals of deficit reduction and a smaller federal government.

ORGANIZATION OF THE BOOK

This book examines major mid-life tasks and concerns: work and retirement, economic security and intergenerational relationships with aging parents and adult children. It also provides information on resources in these areas to help individuals and families accomplish these mid-life tasks. Each chapter includes advice on how to tackle issues and needs, with further sources listed in Appendices A and B and the Bibliography. Policy issues and recommendations are found throughout the book.

The organization of the book is as follows: chapter 2 deals with financial and life planning issues including work, retirement and economic security. The next two chapters are concerned with intergenerational issues.

Chapter 3 deals with adult children living at home, and chapter 4 focuses on relationships with aging parents. Chapter 5 is devoted to women at midlife since they play such a central role in family care and their longevity raises concerns about their economic security in later life. The final chapter looks to midlife and emerging issues in the future.

CHAPTER 2

Economic Security at Midlife: Looking for the Good Years

As a result of increased life expectancy, Americans at midlife today are grappling with numerous concerns that were not faced by their great-grandparents. At the turn of the century, most breadwinners expected to work as long as possible. Many died young and their families survived as well as they could. Women worked because of economic necessity, especially if they were single or widowed. Child labor was common, and many parents relied on their children's contribution to the family income.

Mid-life adults today face a very different future with the likelihood of spending many years in retirement. Regardless of family composition or income, one major focus of mid-life Americans is employment, present and future economic security, and retirement planning, topics considered in this chapter. Intergenerational relationships represent another major mid-life focus. Relationships among family members undergo transformations as children reach adulthood and parents begin to show signs of aging. Chapters 3 and 4 are devoted to these concerns.

DETERMINANTS OF ECONOMIC WELL-BEING

The status of Americans at midlife reflects numerous factors, including marital status, family composition, employment status of the individual and other family members, and ethnic or cultural factors. An individual's or couple's employment experience by midlife will play a large role in their current and future economic security. Savings, other assets and retirement income prospects are closely tied to the workers' occupation and income over the course of their working lives. The prospects for dual-worker families may be more favorable if they have been able to save and build up retirement assets.

Working and Seeking Work at Midlife

Midlife is a time for men and women to evaluate their careers and work histories, to look back on their aspirations and objectives, and to assess their success in reaching goals. Some individuals are exactly where they wanted to be at midlife, at the peak of their careers and earning power. Other individuals may be dissatisfied or bored with work and anxious to change jobs or concentrate on hobbies that offer more satisfaction. If they judge themselves unsuccessful at reaching their goals, they may experience a mid-life crisis and decide to make major changes in their lives (Sheehy 1977).

When they compare their prospects to their parents' situation, some mid-life Americans doubt that they will live as well in later life. There is great diversity in individual and family well-being today, and the gap between rich and poor has continued to widen in recent years. Changes in the economy and the nature of work have resulted in crises for workers who never expected to be unemployed after ten, fifteen or even twenty years with a company.

Losing a job is unsettling at any age, but especially so at 40 or 50 years of age. Ironically, although mid-life workers potentially have many years of productive work ahead, they face many barriers to employment. Despite age discrimination laws, some employers avoid hiring older workers, often defined as anyone aged 40 or over. Others do not want to pay retraining costs for workers whose skills may be outdated. A mid-life worker's new job may pay less, since a large proportion of new jobs created between 1991 and 1993 paid relatively low wages (Ryscavage 1995, 2).

Starting over is costly in other ways for mid-life workers. Replacement jobs may have neither retirement nor health benefits (Ryscavage 1995, 1). Additionally, accepting a job for less pay adversely affects workers' retirement benefits and may affect their lifetime Social Security earnings. This economic crisis may come when mature adults need extra resources for their children's college education or perhaps to assist parents financially. Saving for approaching retirement becomes more difficult under these circumstances (Zal 1992, 117).

The Impact of Structural Changes on Workers

Many mid-life workers cannot understand why they face a precarious future, despite doing exactly what they were taught--working hard and doing a good job. They expected employers to reward them for their contributions, just as their parents were. But national and international trends have weakened or destroyed this employer-employee relationship: "The rapid and fundamental changes in the economy have unraveled the pact between employer and employee that prevailed during nearly three decades of post-World War II prosperity" (Graham 1995, B1).

Consequently, while some Americans forged ahead in their careers and received high salaries, bonuses and other lucrative rewards, others have not prospered. In the 1970s, blue-collar workers faced unemployment when plants closed and jobs were eliminated or moved to countries with lower labor costs. In the 1980s, job insecurity spread to those in white-collar and supervisory positions as cutbacks, mergers and other corporate moves eliminated jobs.

During the 90s, as corporate executives rushed to "downsize," euphemistically called "right-sizing" operations, millions of white-collar, professional, and managerial jobs were lost. Men and women in high-paying jobs who thought that they "had it made" were bewildered to be out of work, especially since profitable companies as well as troubled ones eliminated jobs. During the past decade, millions of jobs were lost and large numbers of new jobs in small companies or the service industries offered lower pay and fewer benefits. Instead of enjoying lifetime job security, individuals now expect to change jobs frequently over their work lives. Young adults just starting out are conditioned to expect this uncertainty, but their parents were not prepared for this type of labor market.

Moreover, wages are no longer linked directly to worker productivity or company profitability. Company executives and shareholders benefit from increased productivity but workers often do not (Lowenstein 1995, C1). Because wages have been flat for a decade, many family budgets have not kept up with inflation. President Clinton raised the minimum wage to $4.25 an hour in 1991, the first increase in ten years. The additional increase to $4.75 an hour in October of 1996 and then to $5.25 in 1997 further benefits minimum-wage workers. However, they still will have about 15 percent less in inflation-adjusted purchasing power than in the 1970s (Lav & Lazere 1996).

The Contingent Work Force

The character of jobs has changed as well. During the 1980s and 1990s, the number of temporary and part-time jobs grew rapidly (AARP 1991; IWPR 1995). The term "contingent" refers to workers employed in part-time, temporary and contract jobs. It may also include self-employed workers. The estimated number of contingent workers varies because definitions differ (Larson 1996). Estimates range from a low of 2 million to 19 million workers. Their numbers are growing because more professional and technical personnel are becoming part-time or contract workers, as are blue-collar workers. Thus, contingent work no longer is confined primarily to clerical and secretarial jobs. Lawyers, accountants, scientists and managers are finding jobs as temporary or contract workers.

Contingent workers are hired by companies to replace laid-off workers, or for specific projects to reduce labor costs. Employers like this arrangement because they can "try out" workers without making a long-term commitment. Those who make the grade may become permanent employees.

These jobs usually do not offer the same wages or benefits as full-time jobs. Mid-life workers may lack health insurance and pensions, and their Social Security benefits at retirement may be lower. As a result, more workers may have to rely on public assistance after retirement. Part-time workers also may be disadvantaged when it comes to unemployment benefits. For example, in 1988, only 10 percent of the unemployed who had held part-time jobs received benefits, as opposed to 36 percent of full-time workers (National Commission for Employment Policy 1995, 34). At the same time, however, executives and shareholders are profiting from record earnings in many corporations with bonuses and lucrative stock options, increasing the income gap between the wealthiest Americans and middle- or low-income workers.

Economic Insecurity in the 1990s

Sources of Anxiety

The economic well-being of adults at midlife today is affected by such factors as family composition, educational background and labor force status of adult members. As the foregoing discussion indicates, employment is a major concern at midlife. Families tend to fare best if they have more than one source of income. However, 24 million Americans live alone today, representing one-quarter of all households (Day 1996, 3). Not surprisingly, adults with higher educational or skill backgrounds and full-time jobs with a full range of benefits are better off.

A majority of married couples depend on two incomes for their economic well-being (Dechter and Smock 1994). Women have become "the new providers" (Families and Work Institute 1995). Some families with two earners enjoy an affluent lifestyle characterized by several homes, expensive cars, exotic vacations and other luxuries. Other two-income families struggle just make ends meet with their combined salaries and could not pay the bills with just one wage-earner. Single-parent families and women who are widowed or divorced often have the lowest incomes.

Growing insecurity about jobs and adequate incomes have made many families even more dependent on two incomes. Women contribute a substantial proportion to family income today, about one-third on average, compared to only one-eighth of a married couple's earnings in 1963. They also are contributing more, regardless of total family income. In some low-income families, they contribute about 36 percent of total income (Dechter and Smock 1994). Since women's labor force participation is becoming more like men's, they will contribute substantially to family well-being in midlife and retirement as a result of earnings, savings and pensions.

More women today are the sole supporters of their families. Some women who were working to supplement the family's income suddenly become the main or only breadwinner when a spouse loses his job, becomes ill or is disabled. The transition to primary earner can be difficult for some women, who experience increased stress and anxiety about family security and their responsibility for meeting financial needs (Mahar 1992a). Since women usually earn less than men, the family's income is likely to be reduced substantially.

Families without two incomes have not fared as well. Incomes in traditional marriages with only one worker improved the least during the past thirty years. Even two-income families may struggle when they use a big chunk of family income for child-care and other work-related expenses.

The economic situation for many single parents is even more precarious. Food, housing and child-care costs may account for almost their total paycheck. If they have to buy health insurance, they have even less discretionary income. Low-income families can take advantage of the Earned Income Tax Credit (EITC), so that they keep a little more income (Lav and Lazere 1996). However, attempts are being made to cut the program, even though it has been supported by both Democratic and Republican administrations and recently expanded. Cuts in public assistance and the Medicaid and Medicare programs also will have an adverse effect on poor and low-income individuals and families.

The Status of Baby Boomers Approaching 50

Seventy-six million baby boomers, born between 1946 and 1964, began turning fifty in 1996. How will this large group of mid-life Americans approach retirement? Some reports suggest that they will do as well as or better than their parents (Congressional Budget Office 1993; Giese 1995), while others see dangers ahead. Their retirement will be affected by complex factors: their employment security and savings rates, future housing values, the future status of the Social Security system and inheritances from their parents. Some will have large college tuition bills if they had children later in life; others will support parents who outlive their own resources (Congressional Budget Office 1993; Graham 1995).

Baby boomers "can't escape being part of a demographic bulge in a stripped-down work place" (Graham 1995, B1). Many of them will be underemployed. Unfortunately, they were reaching their peak earning-power years just as management cutbacks grew. Those who are laid off may turn to self-employment or lower paying jobs; others will work at several part-time jobs, perhaps for less pay and fewer benefits than in their last job. Many will not get the generous pension benefits their parents enjoy.

In general, older boomers will be better off than younger ones, since they had a chance to get established before the employment climate changed. The two groups may be pitted against each other in some situations. Younger workers may think that aging boomers should take early retirement to make way for them, but older workers may not be able to afford retirement.

A 1993 Congressional Budget Office study concluded that baby boomers are saving for retirement at about the same pace as their parents did. However, most expect to retire later, just as they married later, had children later and are paying college bills later (Giese 1995, 53). If they plan to retire at age 65, they will have to figure on having enough resources to live at least until age 85 so that they do not run out of funds in their later years.

Women baby boomers approaching retirement are trendsetters. They have longer, less-interrupted work histories and frequently greater income potential than their mothers did. Their work histories suggest pension benefits closer to those of men and single women (O'Rand, Henretta and Krecker 1992, 82). Since they can expect to live longer than male baby boomers, they will need to accumulate more resources. Retirement planning will be especially important for single or divorced women. (See chapter 5 for a discussion of issues and priorities for mid-life women.)

IS LIVING WELL IN RETIREMENT BECOMING MORE DIFFICULT?

As indicated above, midlife is a time when individuals and couples take stock of their economic status, assessing how they have fared, and determine where they want to be at retirement. Both societal and personal factors play a role in determining an individual's or family's well-being in retirement. National factors, which were discussed above, include the economy and government programs. Major changes in Medicaid, Medicare and Social Security being considered by the Congress and the president may mean that future retirees' benefits may be less than those enjoyed by current retirees. Retirement-age workers may delay retirement in the face of such uncertainties. However, attempts to curb funding for programs to benefit the elderly have met with organized resistance.

Moreover, attitudes toward retirement are being modified, partly as a result of the changes in work and careers discussed above. Retirement is becoming a more ambiguous stage of the life course as individuals move in and out of the labor force, rather than leaving for good (Hayward and Liu 1992, 46; O'Rand, Henretta and Krecker 1992).

Ensuring a comfortable retirement certainly involves planning today. In the past, a secure retirement often was the reward for a lifetime job with one employer. For example, in the area where I live, succeeding generations of a family counted on getting a secure job with generous work and retirement benefits at a major local corporation. Their chances were improved by having relatives employed by the company. This expected scenario changed dramatically in the 1990s, when the company laid off thousands of workers and curbed benefits. The lucrative early retirement packages are gone or scaled down. Job security is no longer guaranteed. This is an example of the changing relationships between companies and employees.

Young adults today find it difficult to think ahead to retirement, when they cannot even find a full-time job. Even workers approaching midlife may not contribute enough to pension plans or save for retirement in the face of mortgage payments, children's education and health care costs.

An important change for workers is the move away from defined benefit retirement plans, which promise a specific pension, to defined contribution plans. In the latter type, such as 401(k) plans, employees get what is in their account when they retire. With these plans, employees are more responsible for planning and contributing to their own retirement, sometimes with employers matching a percent of that amount. How many workers will make retirement saving a priority? Will they make wise investment decisions? Will future retirees have the funds they need, or will they have to take any available job for income and health benefits?

The consequences of these corporate policies will not be seen for years. Since workers also have more responsibility for investing their retirement funds and more alternatives to choose from, they need to make informed choices. They may be unprepared to make decisions affecting their financial well-being because they do not understand their options and the consequences of their decision. Some companies are concerned about whether employees are planning adequately for retirement and are trying to educate them about different types of investments and the risks associated with them.

At the same time, many Americans are affluent at midlife and looking forward to a comfortable retirement. They have sizable pensions, investments and an accumulation of assets like homes, second homes and other valuable property. They need not worry about outliving their assets and may be more concerned about protecting their wealth through tax-saving strategies, estate planning and setting up trusts for their heirs.

Life Choices in Retirement

Individuals and couples at midlife also think about how they will spend their time when careers or jobs are not central interests. What will life after work be like? All that free time can be seen as an opportunity or a cause for alarm. For those with successful careers, the prospect of retirement may be unattractive. Their status and self-image are closely tied to their work. Other mid-life adults can continue to work after retirement, either as independent practitioners, consultants or volunteers. Still others will leave the work force with no regrets and concentrate on other interests. The differences may depend largely on their commitment to work, their success and their interests aside from work. A major hobby, volunteer work or a small business started before retirement might make some eager for retirement. They can move on to something new. Others may take up postponed activities, such as pursuing a college degree or learning a new skill.

Spouses also have to make adjustments to spending more time together. Some look forward to traveling and spending time with family members. However, existing tensions between spouses may be exacerbated by more time together and mutual decision-making. Women who have considered the home their area may find it more difficult to have their spouse "under foot" all day and to have to change their daily routines. Men and women whose social lives have centered around co-workers may miss this familiar social interaction.

Deciding When to Retire

Various economic and social factors influence the retirement decisions of an individual or couple. Obvious aspects to consider are health of the partners and familial obligations, including children at home, grandchildren to raise or elder care needs. An individual's attitude toward work and retirement, as well as perhaps chances for part-time work or a second career, also may be important.

Financial status and resources for retirement living are the most important criteria used by many individuals and couples in deciding when to retire. Retirement income usually comes from three major sources: Social Security, pensions, and savings and/or investments. In the past, retirement planning has reflected "a male-oriented model of retirement timing and retirement income" (Szinovacz, Ekerdt and Vinick 1992b, 259). The amount of Social Security payments at age 62 or 65 often determined when many men retired.

Today's mid-life couples are likely to have two earners. However, these spouses may be at different stages in their careers and have different timetables when it comes to retirement. Women who left the labor force to raise children and then returned to work may be committed to advancing their careers, while their spouses may be contemplating leisure activities in retirement. Consequently, these couples may find their timetables "out of sync," a particular problem for men nearing retirement who are married to younger women at mid-career stages and not interested in retirement (Pollock 1996, A1, A12). In some cases, wives may continue in the labor force while their spouses become "househusbands," taking over some household functions (Gabor 1995).

The retirement decision is becoming a joint one because women spend almost as much time in the work force as do their male counterparts. They also are becoming more empowered by their education, careers and wealth. Therefore, to focus on retirement as determined primarily by male earners, with the females considered "appendages to their husbands," is inaccurate (Hayward and Liu 1992, 24).

With dual-worker couples, numerous patterns of retirement are possible. Brubaker (1985, 31-32) describes the following patterns: the traditional pattern of a single retirement when only the husband works; or "dissynchronized types" in which the husband retires before the wife, usually because he is older and reaches retirement age first, or a rarer pattern in which the wife retires before her husband.

Recent Bureau of Labor Statistics figures indicate that more than one-half of married women, aged 55 to 59 are in the labor force, as are almost one-third of married women aged 60 to 64. Some married women continue to work because they enjoy their work and may want to increase their assets at retirement. Keeping their employer-provided health insurance also may be a motivating factor. On the other hand, single women whose labor force participation mirrors that of men may retire at or near normal retirement age.

Some unmarried, divorced or widowed women may continue to work past the usual retirement age because they cannot afford to retire.

Diverse Circumstances at Retirement

For many, the transition from work to retirement is not final. As Hayward and Liu (1992, 46) point out, "there often is a revolving door between full retirement and part-time work." Some workers in their 50s accept early retirement offers but return to the labor force, either for economic reasons or because they feel too young to stop working. Others cannot afford to retire and work for health insurance benefits or to supplement meager or non-existent pensions. At the time of retirement, the gulf between the wealthiest and poorest segments of society is especially apparent, with some households possessing few resources (CBO 1993; Malveaux 1993; OWL 1995).

The 1993 Congressional Budget Office study of baby boomers' retirement prospects paints an optimistic assessment of their retirement years. It predicts that they will live as well as their parents with some of the same advantages--good lifetime earnings, high Social Security benefits and pension coverage, medical expenses paid in large part by government, and housing appreciation (CBO 1993, 31). Additionally, many will benefit from investment growth over time and inheritances from parents (CBO 1993, 44).

However, the report's authors also underline the contrast between the economic well-being of families with two highly educated earners and the struggles of low-income families with one earner who has less than a high school education and may be unemployed at times. The family is unlikely to own a home, which historically is an important source of capital appreciation. These individuals and families may face an insecure economic future (CBO 1993, xiii).

Another recent study (Smith 1995) found that Americans in their middle and older years have fewer assets than expected. The contrast between the $650,000 in assets owned by the top five percent of white retirees and the lack of any private financial assets for 40 percent of black and Hispanic households is striking. The poor and near-poor in their later years live on only Social Security, perhaps with the addition of Supplemental Security Income (SSI) and food stamps. They have no financial assets, are unlikely to have owned a home, and may have no private pensions. Cuts in government programs may increase the number of poor elderly Americans, a group whose poverty levels dropped in recent decades with increases in Social Security and the introduction of Medicare.

Given these issues and trends affecting Americans at midlife, how can individuals plan for employment security, economic well-being and retirement? The suggested steps listed below represent a starting point. The Bibliography and the resources listed in the Appendices provide more in-depth information and advice on specific topics.

ASSESSING YOUR ECONOMIC STATUS: SOME PRACTICAL SUGGESTIONS

Work and Career Issues

An important goal for mid-life workers is likely to be continued advancement on the job or ensuring that they have a job until retirement, depending on their circumstances.

Increasing Your Chances to Stay Employed

Mid-life workers have no guarantees of working as long as they want or making a smooth transition from work to retirement. They are also more responsible than ever for their own economic well-being in retirement. However, experts suggest the following ways to improve your chances for having and keeping a job:

- Be willing to change jobs or careers if your present situation looks insecure.
- Network with others in your field and with friends and acquaintances to increase your chances of hearing about new opportunities. An executive search firm estimated that about 50 percent of the individuals listed in its data base were currently employed but considered the service as "career insurance" (Graham 1995, B10).
- Keep your skills current and, better yet, increase them or develop skills in a new area of interest. Go back to school, if that is an option, especially if your employer offers reimbursement.
- Take advantage of career-related services offered by your employer to increase your employability. These possibilities include management training programs, skill development courses and seminars, as well as college courses. For example, if you are given the opportunity to learn new technologies, take it. The more diverse and up-to-date your skills, the better your chances of being hired elsewhere if your current job ends. Surprisingly few employees take advantage of opportunities for tuition reimbursement by employers.
- Consider setting aside money to pay for learning additional skills if your employer does not offer such a program. Experts suggest that this step pays, even if you are nearing retirement.
- Don't forget to check whether you are fully vested in your tax-deferred 401(k) plan before making a job change, because you will forfeit part or all of your employer's contributions if you leave too soon (O'Connell 1996, C1,16).

Finding a New Job

These steps can help:

- Take advantage of outplacement services offered by your employer. A growing industry has developed to provide support for terminated employees, including resume writing, interview coaching, office space and facilities. Although questions are raised about how successful these placement efforts are, the services help laid-off workers set up a schedule, have a place to go, and offer information on the job market. At the very least, they provide support and will help you get oriented to job hunting.
- Don't hide in your home because you are embarrassed about being unemployed. Unemployment is common enough today that the stigma is gone, according to experts. Moreover, getting out and meeting others often results in job leads, referrals and suggestions about finding a job. Isolation is the worst course under these circumstances, and can lead to depression and other problems.
- Consider whether you could improve your job hunting by taking courses to broaden your skills or by changing fields if opportunities in your current field are limited. Map out a strategy for either alternative.
- Think about starting your own business if you have the idea, skills and resources to get started. Many new businesses are started under these circumstances. This option could be especially attractive to those taking early retirement. But be careful about tapping into your pension funds for start-up, since the majority of new ventures fail and you might have difficulty replacing that money.
- Don't rule out a less attractive alternative, like part-time work; it might lead to a full-time job. A job paying less than the one you had previously might be worth considering if it offers advancement potential. You might be much better off in six months or a year than if you waited for the better offer that never came. Some job counselors advise volunteer work as a way to increase contacts and experience, and it could lead to a paid job.
- Roll over your pension into an IRA if you leave a job. Don't take the check and blow it. Tap into your nest egg only in a real emergency. Remember how long it took to build it up and how much time you have until retirement.

Getting Help

Networking with friends, colleagues and acquaintances can turn up attractive job leads. Keeping in touch with colleagues also reminds them to call you when they hear of openings. At the same time, don't overdo this tactic or you might find that your calls aren't returned.

Numerous formal and informal sources for job-hunting help exist in your community, including: public employment services; dislocated worker programs; unions, professional and trade associations in your field; community organizations and local networks for unemployed workers. Forty-Plus, a support group for unemployed white-collar executives and professionals, has branches in many cities. Private employment agencies may have job listings in your field, but be sure you understand who is responsible for the fee if you get a job. Read carefully any contract before you sign it.

Computers offer many ways to tap electronically into job leads (see Appendix B). The Internet is expanding daily. On-line employment opportunities are worth checking out and on-line networking may be helpful, especially if you can relocate. Computers also offer a way to do research on companies of interest before approaching them. Don't forget to check out resources at your local public library. It probably has a job bank as well as resources for getting information about possible employers through industry surveys, registers of companies and so on. New business listings published in newspapers or available from city or county government departments also may turn up some names of potential employers.

Taking Stock of Your Resources at Midlife

This section is written for those without much financial planning and investment experience. Those who want more in-depth information should refer to the resources in the Appendices. It is essential to learn about, and take care of, many financial and estate planning decisions if they were not done before.

Adult children who have not begun to plan may learn what's involved when they help their aging parents with financial and estate decisions. While many older adults have well-organized financial affairs, other adult children find parents' plans and records in disarray. They may get "on the job" experience as they try to untangle their parents' affairs after a health or financial crisis.

The importance of saving for retirement is brought home to many adult children who are stunned by their first experience with the costs of home care, retirement community living or nursing home care. A private nursing home easily costs $40,000 per year or more, depending on the part of the country and the type of facility. Another shock comes from the realization that their parents may outlive their resources or face spending down their assets to qualify for Medicaid when they enter a nursing home (See the discussion in chapter 4).

Getting Started: What You Owe vs. What You Own

The first piece of advice is: don't panic if you haven't thought any further about your financial status than how to pay this month's bills. It is not too late to start putting your affairs in order. You will need to figure out your net worth, income and expenses, and your cash flow. Couples can prepare individual and joint statements. If you are recently widowed, you might want to prepare a "Widowhood Statement" (AARP 1988, 37). If you have not done these exercises before, you might find it helpful to consult worksheets and step-by-step advice in books on financial planning like Quinn (1991) and Savage (1991) or guides put out by the AARP (1988, 1991) and the National Center for Women and Retirement Research. Brokerage firms, mutual fund companies, insurance companies and even your employer may provide forms to use in calculating your net worth. Financial management software like *Quicken* will help you to organize the data. But you are the only one who can pull together and plug the information into those forms. Here are some suggestions:

- Don't procrastinate.
- Get your records together--Social Security estimate, pension records, budget or estimates of expenses, tax records and so on.
- Determine your assets including equity in a house, car(s), furniture, savings, pension, investments and life insurance. Then calculate what you owe: mortgage, car and other loans, credit card debt, children's tuition, if applicable, and any other outstanding bills. Subtracting what you owe from what you own will give you an estimate of your net worth.
- Now figure out your income and expenses. If you follow a budget, then your work is done; if not, determine where your money goes every month. Add up your monthly fixed costs for rent, utilities, transportation, child care and so on. Then subtract the total from your income. Hopefully, there is something left over. That amount will give you an idea of what you might save. To save more, decide where to cut costs. For example, could you spend less on lunches or clothing, have fewer evenings out, car pool or use mass transit to save on travel costs, or postpone a vacation?
- Don't be put off by the work involved or because you think it is too late. Even if you can only afford to save a small amount at a time, do it regularly. Tables and charts in many financial planning books and guides show how a nest egg will grow over time through regular savings and illustrate the power of compounding. If you lack discipline, consider having a set amount taken out automatically from your paycheck and transferred directly into a savings option like a mutual fund.
- Pay down debts as quickly as possible and restrict the use of credit cards if you cannot pay them off monthly. Get credit counseling if your debt is unmanageable. Organizations specializing in this service may be found in most areas. They will help you to straighten out the mess you are in and set up a budget to avoid future problems.
- Take advantage of employer pension benefits, including the popular 401(k) plan. Not-for-profit organizations often have a similar program, called a 403(b) plan. These allow you to save money before taxes. If your employer offers to match contributions, it is even more attractive. If neither spouse has a pension plan at work or if your joint income is

low enough, you can put money into an Individual Retirement Account (IRA). Information on eligibility for IRAs and other types of investments is available from the Internal Revenue Service (IRS), financial advisors, books and financial magazine articles.

- Check out other tax-saving programs at work. One popular one allows you to set aside a specified amount for medical, child-care and other expenses before taxes. The amount is decided before the beginning of each year and is forfeited if it is not used.
- Educate yourself about options for saving and investing money and planning your retirement. Make sure that you are comfortable with your choices in terms of risk and return.
- Be sure that any advice and information you get is reliable and unbiased.

Some places to go for information and advice include: public libraries for books and magazines about financial planning and investing; your employer for information about your pension and other benefits, and options like insurance or educational programs; and government agencies, including the Social Security Administration, and the Departments of Labor and Health and Human Services for information about their programs and benefits.

Another source of assistance is a fee-for-service financial planner who offers advice but does not sell products. Check on a financial planner with the Institute of Certified Financial Planners or the National Association of Financial Advisors, and also ask for references so that you can check whether any complaints have been made against them. Seminars on financial and retirement planning also can be helpful, but they often are given by firms to obtain new business, so beware of sales pitches. Don't be pressured to make an investment without seriously investigating both the investment and the seller. Also be sure that it fits in with your objectives and investment philosophy.

The problem faced by investors today is not a lack of information, but rather the vast amount of available material on financial planning, investing and retirement security, much of which is often contradictory. The quality of this information varies and is often designed to sell a specific product. Evaluate any information in light of the source.

Organizations like the American Association of Individual Investors (AAII), the American Association of Retired Persons (AARP), the Older Women's League (OWL), the Pension Rights Center, to name a few, provide educational materials on financial or retirement planning and pensions.

A tested piece of advice when evaluating any investment opportunity is that if it seems too good to be true, it probably is. Even sophisticated investors can be taken in when they do not do their homework or maintain a critical attitude. The recent Foundation for New Era Philanthropy scandal shows how experienced investors lost large sums of money when they were promised high returns on their investment to increase their charitable contributions (Stecklow 1996, A1, A6). The losers were both affluent individual investors and institutions. There is a saying in the financial business that investors are motivated primarily by fear or greed.

Make sure that you thoroughly understand a proposed investment, the risks associated with it and its suitability in relation to your objectives. Remember that the greater the risk, the greater the reward, and vice versa. If the returns promised are far better than any similar investment, be skeptical. If an investment cannot be explained satisfactorily to you, then think twice about putting money into it. You should be convinced that the investment meets both your objectives and tolerance for risk before you make a commitment. Also beware of investment advisors who pressure you for trading authorization over your account. You are giving up control over your assets and you may pay large commissions and lose all or most of your investment.

Also take into account your time frame. The appropriate investment for money needed for a child's education in five years can be quite different from one for your retirement in twenty. Those in their 20s and 30s, who have a long time until retirement, can afford to be more aggressive and take risks (Kobliner 1996; Willis 1996a). Experts usually counsel investing more conservatively the closer you are to retirement. At the same time, however, some portion of your investments should be geared to growth because people are living longer. Additionally, even though an investment has great potential, it is not for you if its volatility will cause sleepless nights.

Investment possibilities keep mushrooming, with new types of investments and companies selling them competing for investor dollars. The huge amount of money being poured into 401(k) accounts make them a special target. The growth in both the number of mutual fund companies and the types of funds over the past ten years has been phenomenal. If you are considering a fund, some factors to consider include whether to buy a load vs. no-load fund and the fit between an investment and your objective. Your objective might be growth, aggressive growth, capital preservation, income and so on. On that basis, you would decide whether to choose a stock, bond, balanced, income or tax-exempt fund, for example. Within stock funds, additional choices may be made among a blue chip, small capitalization, sector or other fund. Some investors find the choices so confusing that they opt for an index fund--for example, one that mimics the Standard and Poor's 500 Stock Index. Lipper Analytical and Morningstar rate funds according to various criteria, and their reports are available in most libraries or by subscription. Numerous references in the Bibliography provide suggestions for 401(k) investing, including *Fortune* articles by Kuhn (1996a) and McLean (1996).

Some investment advisors warn against a popular practice of switching in and out of funds on a short-term basis in an attempt to "time" the markets. Your timing might be wrong or the costs in terms of taxes and fees might eat into profits. Picking the fund with the best short-term record may not give the best results either. Another approach is to assess performance over three, five or even 10 years. Mutual fund tables in financial newspapers and magazines provide this information.

Americans have wholeheartedly embraced mutual funds in the 1990s, but it is not known whether this fervor will survive a sharp market downturn or a recession. Many young or recent investors have not seen the stock market or their funds go down for a sustained period. There has not been a 10 percent market correction during the current bull market, and the next one may shock stock investors. If large numbers of fund investors decide to sell shares during a downturn, other investors will be adversely affected. Investors also need to monitor their mutual funds over time and be alert to any changes in investment objectives, managers or other factors that could affect performance.

Some investors prefer to invest directly in stocks, rather than in mutual funds. If you have enough money to diversify by investing in ten or more stocks, then you might consider this option. For information about investing in individual stocks, see, for example, Lynch (1989). A low-cost way to invest in stocks is to buy shares directly from companies with Dividend Reinvestment Plans (DRIPS). Otherwise, you might join an investment club and pool your regular contributions with others. You also would have an opportunity to learn about companies and picking stocks (see Beardstown Ladies 1994). Some investment clubs are using high tech tools like the Internet to get information and make investment decisions.

The next section provides more advice about financial planning and investing for retirement.

Where You Are vs. Where You Want to Be at Retirement

If you are ready to find out what it will take to retire with the same lifestyle you are now enjoying or better, get out a pad and pencil or use the prepared tables and charts in books or manuals on financial planning. Numerous retirement planning software programs will take you step-by-step through the process. If you are a computer devotee, you probably have a favorite financial management or retirement planning software program and have already entered data in your computer. Others will have to pull together the information.

This exercise may be anxiety-provoking for some, especially if they have done little preparation. Others may have already filled out spreadsheets listing their assets and made projections of their economic situation at retirement. They also probably keep track of investment performance on an annual and quarterly basis. If you have already figured out your net worth, as suggested in the "Taking Stock" section above, then some of the work is done. Two-earner couples will put together two sets of numbers for their joint future.

If you are using a pen-and-paper approach, the first task is to figure out what you will need to live on in retirement. Experts suggest that you will need about 70-80 percent of your current income after you retire, since some expenses will go down. If you are frugal, you can manage with less. You also may find that expenses will go down after the first few years. Your house may be paid for and clothing, restaurant, and costs associated with work will be eliminated. Of course, expenses for items such as health care, travel, relocation to a warmer climate or to be near children and grandchildren, may go up.

Sources of Retirement Income

Now, figure out the sources and projected amounts of retirement income. Most retirees derive income from three major sources: Social Security and other government income; traditional pensions, 401(k) or 403(b) plans, and Individual Retirement Accounts; other savings and investments. Two assets that many financial advisors suggest *not* including in your calculations are (1) the projected value of your home and (2) a potential inheritance. Predicting the value of your home when you retire is difficult. After the boom years and skyrocketing housing values in the 1980s, some homeowners are finding that their homes are worth less than they paid for them. So if you include your home, be conservative in estimating its worth at retirement. On the other hand, housing can provide you with future income in the form of a reverse mortgage. The costs and benefits of such a step need to be weighed carefully.

As people live longer and nursing home care costs increase, many advisors think that an inheritance from parents or other relatives may become less likely. Smith (1995, 15) found that two-thirds of those in white and 90 percent of those in minority households had not received an inheritance by their mid-50s.

However, individuals still may estimate future money transfers that might occur between generations. Money can flow in several directions. While some mid-life Americans may contemplate inheriting from their parents, others expect resources to flow in the other direction. They contemplate that their nest egg will be reduced by providing financial support to their parents or children.

Subtracting where you are today from where you want to be at retirement will indicate the savings between now and retirement. Dividing that sum by the number of years left will give you a rough estimate of the amount to save annually. Adding an estimated annual return on that investment can give you more at retirement or decrease the amount you need to save. This brief exercise is meant as a way to start figuring out your status. Resources at the end of the book will provide more detailed information. If you cannot complete this task on your own, consult professionals in financial planning for help.

Developing a Plan

When you know where you stand, the next step is to improve your economic well-being in retirement. That may mean increasing your contributions to an existing pension plan or savings. Giese (1995, 53) gives some practical advice: "More is better than less and the sooner you start saving, the better." To boost returns, a change in the mix of investments might be indicated, but keep in mind where you fit on the risk-reward equation. In two-

24 Americans at Midlife

earner families, both spouses should contribute the maximum to their plans, especially if employers match their contributions.

If you are fortunate enough to have a pension plan at work, find out about your options and responsibilities for contributing to the plan. How much can you set aside on a non-taxable and taxable basis? Will your employer match part or all of your contribution? Does you employer have an Employee Stock Ownership Plan (ESOP)? Also be sure that you understand your employer's responsibilities for ensuring that your pension is there when you retire (see Malveaux 1993, 181; Schultz 1996a and b; Johnston 1995). Can it be ended if the company is bought out? Can your employer borrow from it? How portable is your pension? Can you take it with you if you change jobs? How long must you be with the company or organization before you are vested. When you retire, what are your options for receiving your pension? Can you take a lump sum or only monthly payments?

Employers should provide information about retirement plans at least on an annual basis, or more frequently if requested. They also may make projections of an employee's retirement income, including estimated Social Security payments at retirement for long-term employees. To get an estimate of your projected benefit directly from the Social Security Administration, request Form Number SSA-7005-SM-SI. Those who have worked for the same employer a long time may be lucky enough to have a defined benefit plan, and have the option of a regular annuity check or a lump-sum payment at retirement. Others will get the amount in their 401(k) plan at retirement, an amount largely dependent on what they have contributed. Since most employers now are required to offer various options for 401(k) investments, decide what is best for your objectives and situation (see, for example, Spraggins 1995).

If you do not have a company pension, start or continue saving regularly, even if the amount is small. If you re self-employed, do not ignore the importance of setting money aside. The earlier you begin, the greater the benefit from compounding over time. Take advantage of IRA possibilities if you and your spouse meet the guidelines. If you lack discipline, arrange an automatic withdrawal from your checking account.

Couples have to decide who will be responsible for retirement planning and managing investments. If one partner is more interested, experienced or a better saver, then that partner may take on the job. The same decision may be made with regard to money management and saving. Some couples prefer to keep everything separate and manage their own money and investments.

When you change jobs, roll your pension over into an IRA or a new company plan, if that is an option. Do not take possession of the check for two reasons: (1) it will be subject to a stiff penalty for early withdrawal and (2) you might be tempted to spend it. Studies have shown that many workers who receive their retirement money after a corporate buyout spend the money on a new house, car, vacation and so on (Schultz 1995). Some pay off loans or use the money for their children's education. These latter choices may be good uses for the money, but the retirement funds may not be replaced.

Since employees have more responsibility for retirement saving today, educate yourself and make informed choices. A summary of suggestions offered earlier in the chapter includes:

- Learn about the risks and rewards of various types of investments.
- Determine your risk tolerance. If you are worried about losing money, you may want to start conservatively and perhaps gradually take more risk.
- Invest with your specific time horizon in mind. The longer the time till retirement, the more risk you can assume. If you choose only "safe" investments like certificates of deposit (CDs), you will not keep ahead of inflation.
- Be sure that your investments are diversified. All of your retirement savings should not be in company stock, for example. Also, check on your employer's contributions to the account. Some strange and risky items like collectibles have turned up in some pension funds (Schultz 1996a, A1, A8).
- Monitor your 401(k) plan to be sure that it is not being raided or used illegally by your employer (Johnston 1996). If your employer seems to be on shaky ground, find out what will happen if the company goes bankrupt. If the company gets taken over by another, will your retirement money be safe? The Department of Labor monitors the underfunding of pension plans and has been warning some companies to remedy the situation.

Seminars on investing held either at work or in the community can be informative, but always assess recommendations in light of the presenter's background and objectives. Even courses sponsored by non-profit organizations often are given by investment professionals whose goals are new clients. Investment advisors of all kinds are vying for those large lump-sum pension payments being rolled over into IRAs.

Helpful information on retirement planning and pensions is available from the U. S. Department of Labor's Pension Education Department, including brochures on the "Top Ten Ways to Beat the Clock and Prepare for Retirement" and "What You Should Know About Your Pension Rights." The American Association of Retired Persons (AARP) has numerous helpful publications, including *Focus Your Future*. The Pension Rights Center offers numerous publications and telephone advice. A Women's Pension Policy Consortium, composed of the National Senior Citizens Law Center, the Older Women's League (OWL), and the Pension Rights Center, has prepared material for working women concerning their pension rights and needs. Numerous financial magazines and newsletters offer advice, as do videotapes available from many sources. See the Bibliography and Appendices for more information.

Other aspects of financial and estate planning will be discussed in chapter 4 in relation to aging parents. Wills, living wills and powers of attorney are basic documents for any individual and couple to have at midlife, if not before. Such documents are doubly important in families with young children for whom a guardian should be named. Parents also may want to discuss their retirement and estate plans with their children. They will know what to expect and will be prepared in the event of an emergency. Mid-life women and men who have hunted for their parents' records and tried to figure out what they would have wanted are likely to make sure that their own children do not go through the same experience.

CHAPTER 3

Mid-Life Parents and Adult Children: Many Nests Aren't so Empty

INTERGENERATIONAL RELATIONSHIPS AT MIDLIFE

A second set of concerns for mid-life individuals and couples centers around intergenerational relationships. They are adjusting to their children becoming adults and to their parents growing older. This chapter begins with a brief overview of general intergenerational issues, followed by its major focus on mid-life parents and their adult children. Chapter 4 deals with relationships between mid-life adults and their parents.

Mid-life families have been called the "new pioneers" by Shanas (1980) because they may include as many as four or five generations. As Riley (1983) pointed out, we do not know yet how great-grandparents will fit into the kinship structure. New coalitions or interactions may develop among generations. Bonds may be strong or weak. In some families, great-grandparents are honored and occupy a central place in the family. In others, they may be seen as a social problem by relatives and the community because of extensive care and service needs. The middle generation may feel even more squeezed if they assume economic and social responsibility for grandparents (or grandchildren), as well as their parents and adult children.

No role models exist for family members to follow. In the not-so-distant past, children might not even have reached adulthood before both parents died. At midlife today, adults may have two older generations alive. In some families, little contact may occur between the oldest and youngest members, but others have a tradition of huge family gatherings that are attended by all living family members.

Divorce and remarriage further complicate intergenerational relationships. Few guidelines exist for determining who is considered to be a part of the family or what relationships are appropriate for those no longer related by marriage; family members have to work out their own responses to such situations. Some former relatives interact amicably; in other families, ex-relatives may maintain a social distance or display outright hostility.

Grandparents face an especially difficult situation when their children divorce. If their daughter has custody of the children, they may see them frequently. However, if their son or daughter is not the custodial parent, they may have little contact with their grandchildren. Some have sued for the right to spend time with their grandchildren. Relationships with their grandparents may represent important sources of continuity for the children after divorce, especially if parents remarry and establish new households. The children may become part of a blended family and have to work out a new set of relationships.

The strong element of reciprocity in intergenerational transactions sometimes is forgotten. With so much emphasis on caring for ill and fragile aging parents who require considerable support, it is easy to forget that many parents are active and self-sufficient into their 70s and 80s. Moreover, grandparents today are often in their early 50s or even younger. Assistance goes both ways, with older generation members frequently assisting younger ones. They may offer financial help, perhaps assisting with costs of a home mortgage or a grandchild's education (Duff 1996). Parents also provide social support through activities like baby-sitting and child care, planning family gatherings, and invitations to their vacation home. Troll (1989, 219) describes this reciprocity of interactions over a family's lifetime as "flowing more toward younger generations at first and shifting toward older generations as circumstances change."

At the same time, parental roles and responsibilities do not end when adult children leave home. They may help the younger generation get established with money and gifts. Their socialization influence also persists, since children often model their behavior after their parents' behavior. Not only does the parent-child bond continue, it may strengthen over time. So family members establish a complicated web of mutual responsibilities, support and benefits over the life course.

At times, intergenerational relationships create strains for those at midlife, especially when family members suffer from chronic and debilitating illness. It is also not uncommon for unresolved tensions from the past to flare up, often involving siblings as well as parents and children. A crisis may bring out half-forgotten rivalries or resentments. It also may bring family members closer together as they support each other or the one who needs help.

"Sandwiched In"

The current generation of mid-life adults has been dubbed the "sandwich generation." Some argue that the term is not meaningful since to have three generations living in the same household is relatively rare. In fact, few parents over 65 years of age live with their children (Loomis and Booth 1995).

Research also indicates that relatively few mid-life adults who care for aging parents still have children at home (Taeuber 1992; Loomis and Booth 1995). Nevertheless, it seems that the term would be more meaningful if it were used more broadly to refer to mid-life adults who experience pressures and strains from their responsibilities for older and younger generations, whether or not they live in the same house. Mid-life adults with an ill or disabled child and a parent needing care have multiple, perhaps long-term care responsibilities.

Retirement planning may be modified when dependent children or parents need care. Couples may defer a planned post-retirement move to remain near older or younger family members. Adult children or parents may make frequent demands, especially if they are the only relatives close by (Szinovacz et al. 1992b). Such expectations may involve elder care or baby-sitting and other responsibilities for grandchildren. Expected leisure time may evaporate to meet requests for help. Single adult children often feel pressured to stay close to their parents and may bear significant financial burdens for their care.

Cronin and Kirk (1991) studied thirty middle-aged and older persons in the Washington, D. C., area who were helping a parent, spouse or older relative while also providing assistance to an adult child or young-adult relative. The financial costs were clear: average assistance amounted to almost $20,000 for older relatives, mostly for medical and health care costs, while living expenditures represented the major part of assistance to younger relatives.

There also were other costs. Respondents reported refusing job advancement opportunities, incurring debt or liquidating assets, or working fewer hours to meet these responsibilities (Cronin and Kirk 1991, 2). The burdens fell disproportionately on single women. Children or parents were not the only care recipients; these adults also helped in-laws, aunts, cousins, nieces and nephews. The authors described these mid-life and older Americans as the "sandwich generation" or, to use Brody's (1990) term, "women in the middle."

This small study suggests how mid-life adults feel squeezed financially and emotionally. The authors concluded that more financial planning assistance would help these families improve their own and the older generation's economic well-being. Even adults with more education and experience did not know about available resources and often misunderstood programs like Medicare. Dependent young adults also needed money management skills (Cronin and Kirk 1991, 25).

Certain mid-life individuals and couples seem to experience more strain when their life stages and responsibilities are "out of sync" with each other, leading to additional pressures. Some examples of these situations are:

- couples who had children late in life, because of delayed childbearing or second marriages, and face parent care issues at the same time as childrearing;
- parents whose adult children come back home to live while they themselves are caring for their own parents;

- grandmothers raising their own children and their children's children, or raising grandchildren when they looked forward to an empty nest. This arrangement will become more common with cuts in public assistance benefits to teens and the denial of benefits to teens who set up their own households.
- Another difficult situation occurs for women or men with a spouse and an older parent who are ill at the same time. The well spouse may care for the ill relatives and also assume the financial or day-to-day management of two households. Such caregiving for members of the two generations does not occur simultaneously as a rule.

BOOMERANG KIDS: WHO SAYS YOU CAN'T GO HOME AGAIN?

A relatively recent phenomenon in the American family is the increase in young adults living at home. This development changes the conditions of midlife for many parents who expected an empty nest at this stage of their lives. Relationships between parents and their adult children also are changing at this time. In fact, the term "adult children" is an oxymoron, conveying ambiguity in relationships between children and parents at midlife and beyond. These relationships are not exactly between equals, whether in the case of parents and grown children or mid-life adults and their aging parents. The history of earlier relationships lingers.

Attitudes toward this stage in life are changing as well. The impact of the "empty nest" on parents has been reexamined in recent decades. Rather than finding the expected responses of emptiness and concern as childbearing and childrearing ends, researchers have found that parents experience increased marital satisfaction, regardless of the quality of their relationships with their children. This reaction seems related to the fact that a stressful period has ended. It also may reflect the financial relief that parents expect (White and Edwards 1990; Suitor and Pillemer 1987).

Parenting had been regarded as a "time-limited commitment" (Schnaiberg and Goldenberg 1989, 256). Children were expected to leave home around the time of going to college or entering the labor force. But the structural factors noted in chapter 2 make it more difficult for these young adults to become self-sufficient today. Consequently, home is seen as a haven for young adults, even if it is not their living arrangement of choice (Schnaiberg and Goldenberg 1989, 256-257).

When young adults do not leave home, or leave and return, both generations have to make adjustments. Parents who have been enjoying a "calmer, quieter, childless household" may not want to become reinvolved with their children's lives or problems on a daily basis (Bianchi 1987, 2). They may not want the added work of another person in the household. At the same time, adult children face difficulties in resuming the dependent child role after being responsible for their own household and perhaps a family as well. They may not readjust easily to parental lifestyles and expectations. If grandchildren are involved, the stress level rises for all concerned and the adjustment is more difficult.

Earlier parent-child relationships play an important role in such adjustments. Adult children who move back voluntarily are likely to have had good relationships with their parents, but the situation may be different if they return because of economic hardship or interpersonal crisis. For some families, the adjustment may be relatively easy; for others, the going can be rough.

One factor that helps parents get through this experience is knowledge that the arrangement is a "safety net" or temporary solution to a short-term need, perhaps divorce, unemployment or the transition from student to worker (DaVanzo and Goldscheider 1990).

Mid-life adults today worry about their children's future security, whether they live at home or not. Many young adults with college degrees have difficulty finding permanent employment. The problems for young people without a high school education or marketable job skills are even greater. Some may become part of a permanent underclass of the unskilled. Current congressional attempts to cut funds for job training will make a bad situation even worse for those who lack skills and a basic education.

Parents tend to feel obligated to support children financially or to let them live at home until they can afford to set up their own household. About 2.9 million adults received financial help from someone outside the household in 1985. One in five was an adult child living outside the parental home and received an average of $3,755 annually (U. S. Bureau of the Census 1988, 7). Children 21 years or older were likely to get assistance to help them maintain consistent living standards. In fact, Americans between the ages of 45 and 64 were almost as likely to support children (44%) as adults (50%). However, only 7 percent supported both adults and children simultaneously, the so-called "sandwich generation " (U. S. Bureau of the Census 1988, 2).

Parents who assume these additional costs may have to divert money from retirement savings or cut back on vacations and leisure activities. However, financial planners caution against spending retirement savings to support an adult child (Rowland 1991, F16). Adult children grappling with mental health or drug problems may need social as well as financial support. They may have trouble living independently and making their own decisions. A few may require long-term or even life-long financial and social support from their parents. These added burdens may occur just as mid-life adults are becoming concerned about their parents' health and independence, or even their own health.

A Portrait of Today's Young Adults

Who are these young adults, and why are they still in the parental nest? About 48 million young adults between the ages of 18 and 29 make up the "twenty-something generation." A large proportion grew up as latchkey kids, who often were home alone or cared for by surrogates while their parents worked. About 40 percent are the children of divorce (Zal 1992, 67). It is not clear what impact their childhood experiences have on them or their attitudes toward independence.

Young adulthood, roughly defined as the years between 18 and 29 (Zal 1992, 68), is a time for making decisions about work, family and marriage, for establishing families and households. In the past, graduate and professional school students were the most likely ones to remain economically dependent, relying on support from their parents until their late 20s. However, many young people today remain dependent much longer, particularly because of housing costs and other economic considerations. They also are postponing marriage. Only 65 percent of those from 25 to 35 years of age had started their own families in recent years, down from 83 percent in 1960. One interpretation is that the stages of life are being stretched out as a result of longer life expectancy (Alperstein quoted in Estess 1994, 56).

Adult children of all ages are living with their parents. More than one-half of all 18-to-24-year-olds lived with their parents in 1990, compared to 42 percent in 1960. Increased numbers of older adult children also lived with their parents. For example, 34 percent of the 8 million never-married adults in their late 20s lived with their parents (Barringer 1991, 18). About one-half of the adult children living at home never left, including those living with older parents (Crimmins and Ingegneri 1990; Suitor and Pillemer 1988). Those who remain at home may become their parents' caregivers in later years.

These statistics represent an important change in living patterns. Until 1988, "twenty somethings" were no more likely than other recent generations of young adults to move back home. After World War II, young people left home to marry; in the 1960s and early 1970s, they left to attend college; by the mid-1970s, they often left for non-family living, either cohabiting or sharing space with roommates. Low housing costs made this alternative possible. However, those who came of age in the 1980s experienced delayed marriage and poor job prospects. They were not "pulled" to move out by the draft, marriage or college. In fact, fewer were going directly from home to college because of high tuition costs (Goldscheider and Goldscheider 1994, 39-41).

This generation is finding it more difficult to be self-sufficient than their parents did. They are seeking permanent jobs and economic stability in an economy characterized by layoffs, "downsizing" and the spread of temporary work, as discussed in chapter 2. Those with college loans may be unable to afford housing, which accounts for a much larger part of their budget than it did for their parents as young adults. So the "pull" to stay at home is strong in the face of an uncertain job market and high housing costs. The family also provides an important safety net when things go wrong (Goldscheider and Goldscheider 1994, 31).

Convenience is a definite factor in living at home since young adult lifestyles are enhanced by the free space, comfort and other amenities, like housekeeping services, that they enjoy. When adult children do not leave, or leave and return, the additional work entailed falls primarily on the mothers.

However, many parents indicated that they do not mind having their children back home (Otten 1990).

Economics are not the only reason why adult children live at home. Bianchi (1987,12-19) analyzed the characteristics of parental households and found that first-born children are the most likely, and the youngest the least likely, to leave home. A mother's marital status also was a factor. If she were remarried, living at home might be less attractive to them. Not surprisingly, parents' ability to support their children was important. The number of family members in the household also played a role. Young adults tended to move out when there was a crowd.

Cultural factors affect whether adult children live at home as well. A large-scale study of 1980 and 1982 high school graduates on the timing and reasons for leaving home found that that African Americans were more likely than whites to be single when they moved out since many delay marriage (Goldscheider and Goldscheider 1994). On the other hand, Hispanics were less likely than white non-Hispanics to leave home before marriage.

Religion and "family values" also were factors, and adult children were more affected by religion than the researchers had expected. For example, Protestant fundamentalist young adults were the most likely of Christian groups to live at home until marriage--or at least during the six years covered by the study. Graduates of Catholic high schools also were likely to live at home until marriage, while Jews left before marriage with the support of their parents (Goldscheider and Goldscheider 1994, 7, 25). A conclusion of the study was that young people have no clear pattern to follow with regard to the timing and reasons for leaving home. There may be no milestone event like marriage or the draft, as in the past.

Parents who had expected their adult children to leave home, just as *they* had done as youths, may find it difficult to accept their children's dependence. They also may communicate these views to their children, creating tension in the household. In their study of high school students, researchers found that when parents and children disagreed about when the child should leave home, the parents often prevailed. To speed up the process, parents sometimes subsidized their children's move to their own place as a way to "buy" their own privacy (Goldscheider and Goldscheider 1994, 7).

The available options for adult children may not be very attractive: to stay home with the possibility of generational conflict or to go out on their own with limited resources. They may be reluctant to choose the latter course because of uncertain job prospects or possibly transient relationships. Then, if they experience financial difficulties or a relationship breaks up, they may have to return to the nest (Goldscheider and Goldscheider 1994, 31).

Returning to the Nest

It is clear from the Goldscheiders' study and other evidence that adult children *do* go home again. Their reasons for leaving and their relationship with parents when they moved out are important in determining their reception on returning. Temporary returns after college or the military have long been expected and accepted. "Twenty somethings" also are accepted back when a job or relationship does not work out.

But what if they left to be "independent," a motivating factor since the 1950s. Those moves have proved temporary for many. The Goldscheiders found that more than 40 percent of young adults who came of age during the Vietnam War and baby-bust periods returned home. When intergenerational disagreements were not a factor in the departure, coming back home usually was possible for them (Goldscheider and Goldscheider 1994, 25).

Some young adults return to the nest when their relationships change. When young couples divorce, one or both may move back with their parents. Cohabitation and unmarried parenthood also increase the likelihood that young adults will return home after being independent. Single parents may live with parents for economic assistance and help with childrearing. This arrangement occurs frequently in the black community, where extended families are not unusual (Dilworth-Anderson 1993). Many grandparents are raising another generation because their daughters cannot care for them or need help in doing so. (See the discussion later in this chapter.)

Adjusting to Living Together Again

Parents may have a variety of reactions when their adult children are living at home again. They may be dismayed or embarrassed that their children have not "made it" on their own, either in the work force or in marriage, and may blame themselves for unsuccessful childrearing. However, as Schnaiberg and Goldenberg (1989, 262-263) point out, these parents often consider their children's unemployment a private matter. They do not see it in the larger context of a public issue resulting from the structural changes in the economy. Parents also may feel guilt or resentment that their lives will be disrupted.

Parents' attitudes toward their children's return and how they cope may improve or worsen the situation. Possible reactions include a period of continuing and unresolved conflict between family members, negotiation with children to create a situation that all can live with, or physical or emotional withdrawal by parents who obviously are not happy and only tolerate the situation (Schnaiberg and Goldenberg 1989, 253).

An important task facing parents is to define their role in this new situation. Do they revert to their earlier ways of interacting with their now-adult children? Do they work to establish new relationships based more on a partnership between equals? Or do they avoid the issue entirely? Regardless of the alternative chosen, parents still have the upper hand to some extent because they are providing room and board. Even though the generational relationship may be *more* egalitarian, children know they are still in a dependent position and have less power.

If their children are home because of unemployment or a failed marriage, some parents lower their hopes and expectations for them. Well-to-do parents may be the most anxious, since they expected their children to replicate their own success. This problem is not confined to children who return home, since so many young adults today cannot find jobs in the fields for which they are trained. Although some are doing extremely well professionally and financially, others are marking time by waiting on tables or taking other temporary jobs for which they are overqualified while they search for permanent work. Parents may despair that despite even their graduate degrees, they may never get established. The children may not expect to live as well as their parents do, since they will be older than preceding generations when they finally begin to climb a career ladder.

Some parents may be tempted to abandon their children, feeling that they have done their job and now their offspring have to survive on their own. They may not want to be reminded that they have failed at preparing their children for adulthood. At the same time, they want to concentrate on their own mid-life concerns and not divert energy or resources to their grown children.

There seems no perfect solution for parents to adopt, since these options involve tradeoffs. Maintaining strong ties to children may divert parents' "time, money, emotional energy" from their own needs and objectives, especially work and retirement planning objectives. On the other hand, withholding support may weaken the ties between the parents and their children (Schnaiberg and Goldenberg 1989, 257). They may regret such a step as they grow older and want to spend more time with their children and grandchildren. They also may lose support from their children in later life.

Parents whose children move back have adjustments to make. Their daily routine may be interrupted by the comings-and-goings of young adults with erratic hours, especially if they are unemployed. Such living patterns may disrupt the schedules of working parents. The older generation also may resent their children's casual attitude toward being unemployed, or object to their lifestyle or irresponsibility.

The burden is usually greatest on the mother, especially if she works at a full-time job in addition to maintaining the household. Cooking and laundry are just two tasks that involve extra work when adult children live at home. Young men often return home partly for the convenient household services they can enjoy (Gross 1991b). Sometimes children help with household work, but the amount of time and effort varies. Daughters seem more likely to help around the house while sons may do yard work or other maintenance jobs. Divorced women may welcome a son's presence for this type of assistance. Despite the extra work and disruption, parents may not mind having their children home again.

Children with the greatest needs and fewest resources gain the most from returning home. They gain social support as well as the use of their parents' resources (Schnaiberg and Goldenberg 1989, 261). On the other hand, those earning good salaries who do not contribute to household expenses benefit by having more discretionary income for luxury items. If they buy expensive cars or other items that their parents cannot afford for themselves, they may engender resentment.

But living at home is not without its costs for young adults, especially the loss of privacy and independence. Their social lives can be affected by living with their parents (Bernard 1994; Scott 1991). They also may have to recognize that a prolonged period of unemployment or underemployment may put them on a path of downward social mobility leading to postponed marriage and parenthood. If they become depressed about being unemployed and avoid job-hunting, they may need professional help to overcome their anxiety.

Numerous negative consequences for parents include:

- the financial costs of supporting an adult;
- unequal contributions by family members to household costs and work, leading to parent-child conflicts over money or household tasks and arguments about values and lifestyles;
- the adverse impact of another person in the household on marital relationships or on younger children who may resent a sibling's return;
- dissatisfaction with the arrangement, but unwillingness to ask the young adult to leave.

Parental reactions to situations generating stress and conflict may be to attempt to control children's lives. Some parents have even taken the drastic step of selling their large house and moving to a smaller one with no room for the children.

On the other hand, the impact is not necessarily negative, and both generations may benefit. The generations coexist amicably in many families. Friendships and perhaps a new closeness between the generations may develop. Both parents and children may enjoy companionship and better understanding. Mothers and daughters may share activities. Divorced or widowed mothers may be happy to have adult children at home, considering it an advantage not be alone. Sons may help out with heavier tasks around the house and outdoors. There may be economic benefits for both generations as well, especially if their resources are limited.

SUGGESTIONS FOR COPING

Fewer resources exist for parents coping with their adult children when compared to all the books and organizations providing advice to those caring for aging parents. This difference is not surprising, since the issues and needs with regard to aging are more complex and often long-term, resulting in greater stress for caregivers. Most parents know that their children's return is temporary and that they either can "make do" or help them financially to move out if they want to reclaim their own home and personal lives.

As indicated above, staying or returning home may require negotiations between young adults and their parents. Factors to be worked out include the needs of both parties, their financial status, the attitudes of those involved (Bianchi 1987, 20), and the rights and responsibilities of family members.

Experts recommend setting ground rules, and Estess (1994, 58) provides the following examples:

- Children are not to engage in activities at home that their parents disapprove of.
- They are to help with household tasks and to care for their space and belongings. Family members will decide who will be responsible for tasks such as laundry, cooking and cleaning.
- Each generation is entitled to privacy.
- Children are expected to be courteous and let parents know their plans-- for example, informing parents if they will not be home for meals.
- They are expected to contribute to household costs. The amount paid toward expenses may be specified. If children do not have the money to contribute, then they can contribute by being responsible for chores.
- They are to concentrate on getting a job, if they are not currently in the labor force.

In other families, members may decide to negotiate aspects of living together by:

- setting parameters of behavior, space and care if grandchildren are living at home;
- setting time limits on how long adult children are expected to live at home;
- negotiating the assistance that parents are willing to provide to help children establish their own household--e.g., lending money for the security deposit and first month's rent.

This list may be too cut-and-dried for some families whose members prefer a more laisser-faire approach. They may be willing to continue with their own lives without setting up specific rights and responsibilities. Zal (1992, 82) offers some succinct advice and guidelines for dealing with adult children: Give them your support but don't "parent" as much; do what you can to foster their independence, and don't take an "I told you so" attitude. He also recommends that parents adopt a cooperative approach to problems, asking for their children's help and developing an atmosphere of mutual respect.

However, it may be important to address financial issues and responsibilities. For example, does the adult child have health insurance? If not, parents have to decide how to arrange coverage. Liability insurance coverage also may be a good step, if it is not already in place. An umbrella liability policy may be advisable when more individuals are living in the household and driving cars. If parents are providing more than one-half of an adult child's support, they may be claimed as dependents for income tax purposes. A minor point is to decide whether to get an additional phone line. The minimal cost is probably worthwhile to avoid the inconvenience of constant incoming calls and a busy line (Rowland 1991, F16).

Families *do* survive the sometimes awkward and tense period when adult children return home, even if they think they won't. The majority eventually find jobs, get married or get their own place to live, and parents get on with their lives.

However, because children are not living at home does not mean that they do not cause parents concern. They may worry about their ability to support themselves or disagree with their choice of lifestyle, spouse or companion. It may be hard for parents to accept that their children are adults and have a right to their choices in life. Children with serious mental or substance abuse problems may need support as crises or reversals punctuate their lives. In *I'm Still Your Mother,* Adams (1994) offers suggestions about handling issues such as the choice of a spouse or friend, sexual preference or careers. The book also offers a list of organizations that can offer advice on a variety of topics.

Young Children and Older Parents

Some households of mid-life couples have a full nest by choice. These are the couples with young children to raise and educate. In some instances, these are second families; in others, couples decided to have another child after the others are grown (Blumenthal 1996). When spouses have both adult and young children, relationships among the family members have to be worked out.

As the caregivers, women find their lives changed by restarting the cycle of raising young children. They may face the most stress and need for adjustment, especially when resuming childrearing at the age of 40 or more. Some find that childrearing is not as easy the second time around when they are older. Fathers may enjoy this later parenting more. They often spend more time with these young children than they did when their older ones were growing up. Some feel guilty that they were largely absent during their older children's formative years and want to make up for it. First-born children may resent the attention given to this new generation.

PARENTING AGAIN AT MIDLIFE: RAISING GRANDCHILDREN

Others at midlife are taking on the responsibility of raising another generation, perhaps almost from birth. These are the grandparents who thought that phase of their life was finished. About one-half million mid-life and older adults are rearing their children's children in households without a parent present

(Chalfie 1994, vii). This phenomenon cuts across racial, ethnic and income categories. The median age of these caregivers is 57 years, with the majority between the ages of 45 and 64 years of age. However, 36,000 are over 75! We are even seeing instances of great-grandparents (who may be only in their 50s or 60s) caring for their great-grandchildren (Gross 1991a, 18).

In addition, some grandparents who live in multigenerational households may not have full responsibility for childrearing but help out when they live with their children and grandchildren. Still others become foster grandparents to children and assume responsibility for their well-being. In the black community, it is not unusual for a family to raise a child who is not a blood relative (Dilworth-Anderson 1993).

Raising children alone is stressful for grandparents. It often is not a short-term or "safety net" undertaking, although it may begin as such. It can be physically and emotionally taxing for mid-life adults who may have been enjoying an "empty nest."

This unexpected responsibility also may come when mid-life adults are ready to retire on fixed incomes and perhaps tight budgets. If caring for a child is difficult financially, grandparents may have to cut back on their own expenses or defer retirement. Others may quit work to provide care on a full-time basis. The burden falls especially heavily on women; 93 percent of single grandparent caregivers are women (Martin 1991, E6).

Yet this arrangement is becoming more common as growing numbers of young parents are unable to raise their own children for a variety of reasons, including unemployment, mental or physical illness, substance abuse, incarceration, AIDS, child abuse and neglect, divorce or teen pregnancy (Chalfie 1994, 1).

Issues for Grandparents Raising Grandchildren

Many grandparents who begin informally caring for their grandchildren face unanticipated difficulties. A recent study by the American Association of Retired Persons (Chalfie 1994) outlined a range of policy-related problems facing grandparents: obtaining financial assistance or health insurance coverage, gaining decision-making authority and settling legal issues. To a large extent, the issues stem from the fact that these "nontraditional" households fall outside the parameters set by those who make policy and set regulations.

Financial assistance can be essential for grandparents on low or fixed incomes. The two main public sources of income support for grandchildren are Aid to Families with Dependent Children (AFDC) and foster-care stipends. Grandparents are eligible for AFDC because grandchildren are related by "blood, marriage or adoption" and live in the household (Chalfie 1994, 6). But some state-level workers do not follow federal guidelines and deny benefits to grandparents or anyone who is not a parent, and others demand evidence of legal custody, even though this is not required by law. The changes in the welfare system passed by Congress and signed by President Clinton at the end of 1996 may make it even more difficult for grandparents to raise grandchildren. The imposition of time limits on public assistance will mean financial hardships for many grandparents if the rules are applied to them.

A better option for grandparents may be foster-care stipends, which are two or three times greater than AFDC payments. However, the qualifying process takes time and entails an invasion of privacy. State requirements also differ. Some states provide grandparents and other related caregivers with payments comparable to those made to unrelated foster parents. However, states are not *obligated* to provide foster-care payments to caregiver relatives. Some state representatives also do not tell informal caregivers about entitlements and helpful services like "psychological counseling, a clothing allowance, and child-care assistance" (Chalfie 1994, 8). Low-income households also may qualify for food stamps. However, some grandparents do not want or need governmental assistance and use their own savings to meet their grandchildren's needs.

Health care coverage represents a major hurdle for many grandparents. Even some employer-provided health care will not cover grandchildren, especially without court-ordered custody. If they do not have private insurance, caregivers may qualify for Medicaid coverage either because of financial need or because they receive AFDC or Supplemental Security Income (SSI). Other grandparents have no alternative but to purchase expensive private insurance for their grandchildren (Chalfie 1994, 8-9).

Decision-making authority is another problem for grandparents without a legal relationship like temporary custody or guardianship. They may be surprised to have trouble enrolling their grandchildren in school or getting school records. They also may lack the authority to make needed medical-care decisions for their grandchildren. For example, crack babies and children with other disabilities may need a guardian's consent for specialized treatment. Grandparents also may need help in dealing with their grandchildren's emotional scars (Martin 1991, E6; Malcolm 1991).

Narrow definitions of the family may give rise to legal issues in other areas such as immigration policy, tax policy and employer leave policies. Recent legislation may make grandparents' responsibilities a little easier. The Family and Medical Leave Act allows grandparents some time off for child care. Another program advantageous to grandparents is the Earned Income Tax Credit (EITC) for which low-income households qualify. With low incomes and an additional dependent, grandparents may be eligible for this benefit. Grandparents also qualify for "head of household" deductions on their taxes.

Ethel Dunn, a founder of the National Coalition of Grandparents, does not think that grandparents who assume the responsibility of raising their grandchildren should have problems because public policies do not recognize nontraditional households. To remedy the situation, she has called for laws to legitimize the multigenerational family (Crowley 1993, 16-17).

In addition to these issues, grandparents need advice and support in adjusting and coping with stress from these new roles and relationships. They may suffer from fatigue, isolation and lack of a social life. They may need respite care at times, just as those caring for aging parents do. For example, women who have children in their 40s often suffer from backaches just from the lifting and bending that they must do. Grandparents in their 60s probably find this type of exertion even more difficult. They also may have major health problems. When her brother died, Liz Carpenter (1994a and b) gave the children from his second marriage a home, despite her own serious health problems and age. She has described the numerous problems and issues she faced and how she managed her unexpected family.

There are economic as well as social costs to taking on such responsibilities. Women may have to decline a promotion or cut back on their hours of work because of child care responsibilities and these decisions may be costly for their own economic security. Grandparents may not only defer planned vacations, moving to another location or leisure-time pursuits, they also may have to postpone retirement because of the costs of raising grandchildren.

Grandparents may have additional worries because of their adult children's difficulties. Such problems as addiction, mental health problems or incarceration may mean that they are unable to spend time with their offspring. Some grandparents have had to bar their children from their home or from contact with the grandchildren because of addiction, child abuse or mental illness. These are difficult decisions for grandparents and may cause unhappiness for their grandchildren. It is difficult for grandparents to accept the possibility that their adult children may not be able to function adequately enough to be parents.

Life is "out of sync" for these adults in their middle years as they begin again to raise children, a chapter in their lives they thought was over. Other grandparents find their lives out of sync because they are raising their teen-aged children's children and their own younger children in a home that may be too small for three generations. With too many family members crammed into too little space, the potential for conflicts or just getting on each others' nerves is multiplied. Noise from children playing or from loud music may be especially distracting for the older generation.

Help for Harried Grandparents

Help does exist for grandparents. Their circumstances are being recognized by organizations like the AARP and support groups across the country. However, they will need to seek out the information and help they need. They will have to apply to agencies of the federal, state and local governments to obtain benefits to which their grandchildren are entitled. If they are uncomfortable with the thought of facing bureaucratic representatives, they may want to find informal support groups to get a quick orientation on where to start and how to prepare for meetings with agency representatives. Such groups can tell them about the paperwork needed, questions to ask and reactions to expect. They also can give them an idea of how long the process will take.

Many local organizations and agencies provide information and services. Each community has its own groups, as well as branches of state or national organizations. A local support group can provide valuable assistance by steering grandparents to the right places and offering time-saving tips. Support groups or networks also offer an antidote to isolation, an outlet for anger or frustration, and ideas for coping with parenting (Smolowe 1990).

Information and assistance also can be obtained from social organizations for children and families, churches, religious or grassroots neighborhood groups. The yellow pages of the telephone directory or a city or county human services directory provide a starting point in locating organizations. The local bar association, legal services offices or law clinics can provide information on custody, guardianship and adoption assistance.

The state or county Department of Social Services, local or state public health offices, or community health clinics will provide information on medical care; the local Department of Social Services on financial assistance; and local mental health associations and support groups on counseling or support for caregivers and the grandchildren.

If grandparents are not sure where to start, several national groups will link caregivers to referral services. For example, the AARP has prepared numerous reports and helpful hints, available from:

AARP Grandparent Information Center
Call (202) 434-2296, weekdays from 9 a.m. to 5 p.m. or write to:

AARP Social Outreach and Support
601 E Street, NW
Washington, DC 20049

For information on a support group near you, these organizations can help:

ROCKING (Raising Our Children's Kids: An Intergenerational Network of Grandparenting)
P. O. Box 96
Niles, MI 49210

Grandparents United for Children's Rights
137 Larkin Street
Madison, WI 53705
(608) 238-8751
This organization works with grandparents seeking more access to their grandchildren.

GAP (Grandparents as Parents)
P.O. Box 964
Lakewood, CA 90714
(310) 924-3996

CHAPTER 4

Children and Parents: Aging Together

MYTHS AND REALITIES ABOUT AGING

The increase in life expectancy during the twentieth century helps to explain mid-life Americans' focus on the well-being and care needs of their parents. The "graying of America" is evident everywhere, from the barrage of articles, commentaries, and advertising directed toward the growing number of people aged 65 and over to concerns about the uncertain status of Social Security and rising medical care costs for older Americans. The competition by brokerage houses, insurance companies, mutual fund companies and financial advisors for the assets of retiring workers and affluent older people testifies to the economic importance of this segment of the population.

Older Americans also have plenty of political clout. Politicians seem unwilling to antagonize those who are 65 or older, as demonstrated by unsuccessful government efforts to curb Medicare costs and modify the Social Security system to keep it solvent. Aging Americans have a powerful interest group in the American Association of Retired Persons (AARP), which advocates effectively on behalf of its large membership. In contrast, opposition to cuts in welfare spending at the state and federal levels has been less organized and much less successful. Young children, the primary beneficiaries of public assistance and related programs, have few organized groups to speak for them or protect their interests. [Perhaps to remedy this imbalance, the Children's Defense Fund (CDF) organized a 1996 Washington march to demonstrate support for children's needs and interests.]

Statistics reveal an aging U. S. population. According to the 1990 Census, 31.1 million Americans were 65 years or over, representing 12.5 percent of the population. They also are living longer. Almost 7 million were 85 years or older and about 36,000 were 100 years or over, double the number in 1980. Women continue to live longer. Seventy-nine percent of this "oldest of the old" group, those over 85, was female (Taeuber 1992, 5). Projections are that this fast-growing group will reach nearly 17 million by the year 2050, indicating that elder care will be a growing issue in the next century (Taeuber 1992, 2-5).

The older American population also is becoming more diverse as greater numbers of blacks and Hispanics live into their 80s or older. There also have been relatively large increases in the older population of Asians, American Indians and Hispanics (Taeuber 1992, 2-9, 10). The life expectancy for minorities, however, is still less than that for whites (Taeuber 1992, v).

The economic well-being of older individuals also varies. Many magazine articles and television commercials portray the affluent lifestyle of 65-and-over Americans who live in luxurious retirement communities in the Sun Belt, travel widely and enjoy a high standard of living. Other older Americans enjoy a modest but comfortable retirement. Government-assistance programs like Medicare and Social Security, coupled with generous pension benefits and home ownership after the Second World War, have meant a secure retirement for many. Yet others are not so fortunate, and many older Americans live in poverty or near poverty in their later years.

In recent decades, poverty has decreased significantly among older Americans. Only 12 percent of the elderly, compared to 23 percent of children, were classified as poor by the Census Bureau in 1993. Without Social Security and other government payments, however, one-half of those 65 years and over would be poor (Treas 1995, 23-24). Medicare, food stamps and subsidized housing also improve the lives of older Americans. Yet many older Americans still are trapped in lives of near-poverty. In stark contrast to the picture of well-to-do seniors enjoying their retirement years is the plight of the 43 percent of elderly black women living alone who are classified as poor. Others with incomes just above the poverty level in 1993 were barely managing; a major health or economic reversal would push them into poverty (Treas 1995, 26). Even those with a house or other assets may have little available cash for daily living expenses or the health care costs not covered by public or private programs.

On an individual and family level, these demographic changes translate into mid-life adults' concerns about the economic, social and health status of aging family members. They have to come to terms with their parents' aging, potential loss of independence and eventual death. Adult children who help parents make decisions about living arrangements, financial matters and health care are likely to wonder about their own futures. However, the picture need not be gloomy. Many older individuals are healthy and independent. Moreover, this generation of mid-life Americans is trying to improve its chances of staying healthy and active in later life by eating sensibly and exercising regularly.

This chapter provides a review of aging issues from the adult children's perspective and suggests approaches to working with parents on financial and caregiving needs. Mid-life adults who want in-depth advice about parents and aging can consult the Bibliography and Appendices for topics of interest. Sources listed include first-person experiences and advice, as well as organizations and support groups for further information. It also should be noted that, although the focus is adult children and their aging parents, the discussion is equally relevant for mid-life adults caring for other aging relatives or friends. The chapter ends with a look at some policy issues.

Other topics not discussed here are covered in numerous books on aging parents. For example, Zal (1992) offers advice for children with a parent who is at a loss after retirement or the death of a spouse. He also discusses the conflicts that come about when children and parents have differing views about the nature of retirement. Children may expect their parents to be more active than they themselves want to be.

Some Myths

Many myths about aging or parent-child relationships in later life are contradicted by research and anecdotal evidence. Some prevalent ones include the following:

- **All aging parents lose their independence and need care**. There is great variability in the health of older Americans. Adults in their 60s, 70s and even 80s often are healthy and involved in many activities. Many are independent until a final short illness and never require extensive care (Friedan 1993; Riley 1983). Some may need only periodic advice and emotional support from family and friends. Others eventually need assistance with daily living or even total care. However, only 5 percent of Americans over age 65 are in nursing homes at any one time, a statistic that is surprising to many.

- **Aging involves an inevitable deterioration of abilities,** as evidenced by memory loss, inability to change, helplessness and preoccupation with death. We all know people in their 80s and 90s who disprove this view. Examples of individuals who remained active and productive at advanced ages include the Delany sisters (1994); Barbara McClintock, the scientist who won a Nobel Prize for her discoveries only after a lifetime of work; and culinary expert Julia Child, who is still active. Marjorie Stoneman Douglas continued her work to preserve the Everglades after she celebrated her 100th birthday. Many men and women in the arts have continue to work even though they are well past normal retirement age. Some who come to mind are actors George Burns and Jessica Tandy, the director George Abbott, photographers Berenice Abbott and Henri Cartier-Bresson, and the artist Georgia O'Keeffe.

- **Intergenerational assistance only flows from adult children to aging parents.** The theme of reciprocity between the generations is especially relevant to parent-adult child relationships. Aging parents often help their children with major expenses like buying a house or grandchildren's tuition. They provide emotional and financial support to adult children, especially during crises like divorce or unemployment (Troll 1989). Aging parents also may feel weighed down by their adult children's problems, rather than the children worrying about their parents (Pillemer and Suitor 1991b). Young and old also help each other when a family member is ill.

- **When generations live together, adult children do all the work and provide all the services.** Intergenerational households composed of adult children and their parents are relatively rare. However, such households may achieve a better standard of living for members by sharing expenses and resources. This arrangement may especially benefit low-income single parents who also get help from the older generation with child care. Intergenerational households are more common among various ethnic groups, including Asians, blacks and Hispanics (see Dilworth-Anderson 1993; Barresi and Menon 1990; Brubaker 1985, 54).

- **Caring for aging parents is always a financial drain on adult children.** There is considerable debate on this issue, probably because the economic status of older persons varies. Far from needing help, some older Americans begin to transfer wealth to their adult children and grandchildren during their lifetimes, perhaps by helping the children purchase a house (Englehardt and Mayer 1994). The likelihood of an inheritance varies, however, and is rare among blacks (Bumpass and Aquilino 1995, 28). Moreover, since some older individuals barely have enough resources for their own needs, financial assistance may flow from children to parents. Poor elderly Americans may have to rely on their families or on government assistance to survive.

PLANNING WITH PARENTS FOR THE FUTURE: MAJOR TASKS

When adult children reach midlife, their parents may be economically independent, healthy, and still working or enjoying retirement. Yet by their mid-to-late 40s, at least one-half will have a widowed parent who may need help. At this stage of life, the adult children's circumstances will vary as well. Given the tendencies toward later marriage, divorce, remarriage and later childbearing, sandwich-generation members may be grappling with the illness or death of a parent while they still have young children; others will be retired by the time their parents die (Bumpass and Aquilino 1995, 19-20).

When parents need care in their later years, adult children may increase their assistance gradually. Caregiving responsibilities also may arise suddenly after a parent has a heart attack, stroke or other major illness. With parents living longer, adult children may be in their 60s or older, when caring for ill or frail relatives is more difficult. With more four-generation families, mid-life adults may have grandparents as well as parents who require care (Taeuber 1992, v).

When Parents and Children Live Apart

Geographic mobility makes interaction between adult children and parents more difficult. Adults at midlife may live far from their parents because of job opportunities or mobility (see Bumpass and Aquilino 1995; Climo 1992). In some cases, aging parents are the ones who move, choosing to live in warmer climates after retirement. Some will move again as they age, perhaps to be nearer to their children. Research indicates that those with more education are likely to live farther away.

If family members live in different parts of the country, children may worry about whether their parents are managing well or getting the assistance they need. With telephone contact, parents can withhold important information about their status, worries or recent crises. They may not want to alarm their children about failing health or admit to difficulties in daily living. It is important to listen as carefully for what they *don't* say as what they do. If other relatives live near the parents, they can provide first-hand information about their status. Needless to say, when parents require daily living assistance, children who live nearby are likely to assume primary responsibility for their care, in consultation with siblings or other close relatives.

If no relatives live near the parents, then distant children may either supervise such care from afar or hire a geriatric care manager to do it for them. This recent specialization developed because so many families are scattered across the country today and cannot provide or monitor a relative's care. Moreover, when both the husband and wife work, they have less time to make frequent trips back and forth to verify that arrangements are working satisfactorily. If adult children supervise care from another city, they will need to check thoroughly the references of those they hire and to designate someone in the area to monitor the situation on a regular basis.

All intergenerational relationships do not occur over long distances, however. Bumpass and Aquilino (1995, 22) found that about one-half of adult children aged 40 to 44 live within 25 miles of their parents and about one-third see them weekly. About 40 percent of those with a living parent see them weekly throughout midlife. Another interesting research finding is that children in larger families tend to live closer to their parents (*Wall Street Journal* 1994, B1).

Tackling Difficult Topics

As parents age, their children may face making emotion-laden decisions with them about financial and estate planning, living arrangements, and assistance with daily living or comprehensive care needs.

Financial and Estate Planning

Adult children almost always find discussing financial and estate planning with parents difficult, since they involve "two of our culture's three big taboos--death and money" (Sharon Rich quoted in Asinof 1993, C1). A specific event or crisis may serve as the trigger for the discussion. If parents are considering a change in living arrangements, they may want to put together financial data to assess the economic feasibility of moving versus staying. If they are contemplating an assisted care facility, they probably will have to prepare a detailed financial statement as part of the application process. A parent's illness may make a discussion about finances crucial, but it may be too late to get information from them. The title of Asinof's (1993) article says it all: "The Talk You Must Have with Your Parents." These matters are best decided when parents are in good health and clear about their wishes, rather than after a health crisis when they may be unable to make their preferences known. Clements (1995a) approaches this difficult topic in the form of a letter to his parents.

Willis (1995) outlines some basic steps to ensure that parents or other aging relatives will receive adequate care in their later years: get the facts early, make plans for living expenses and protect against major long-term illness.

Of course, some older persons already have taken care of estate planning and put their finances in order. In fact, they may be urging their children to do the same. Other older persons procrastinate and avoid making the difficult decisions. Everyone knows an older person who alternately berates and cajoles younger family members with promises or threats about who will get what and why in their will.

Basic steps: Although it is beyond the scope of this book to provide detailed financial and estate planning advice, certain basic steps are needed. Adult children and their parents should take care of the following matters:

- information about current income and sources--Social Security, pension, investment income, annuities, individual retirement accounts (IRAs), etc.;
- a will;
- a durable power of attorney;
- a health care proxy;
- a list of assets, the location of the paperwork, and the names of people to contact, including brokers, insurance agents, lawyers and account numbers. Some survivors spend months looking for belongings stashed in unlikely places by aging parents. Some books and organizations provide convenient forms for organizing this information. A computer record is especially handy to have since it can be easily modified as circumstances change.
- information about health insurance and a consideration of whether long-term health care insurance makes economic sense;

- additional important documents, including a living will and a letter of instructions about disposition of personal belongings;
- funeral instructions, which are an even more difficult subject to discuss with parents. Some individuals write a letter specifying their wishes. Without such information, surviving relatives must decide what they *think* the person would have wanted.

The importance of putting one's house in order increases when parents have remarried or when their children have divorced and remarried (American Institute for Economic Research 1995). The potential for conflicts and haggling among survivors is multiplied when aging parents have not made their wishes known (*Sandwich Generation* 1996). Some parents will have made prenuptial agreements or set up trusts for children and grandchildren from current or previous marriages.

Decisions in these sensitive areas are understandably threatening to aging adults for several reasons. First, they are reluctant to give up their independence prematurely, especially control over their assets by granting power of attorney to another person. This concern exists even when such control would be ceded only if they became incapacitated. Second, since older individuals may fear outliving their resources, they may worry that their children might take risks with their assets. Nevertheless, an adult child (or other relative) probably should be designated to act for parents concerning financial matters in an emergency (Willis 1995).

But those whose assets will last a lifetime are the lucky ones. They have alternatives if they cannot manage in their own homes. Low-income families have limited options and may rely either on care by relatives, perhaps in an extended family arrangement, or a nursing home if they need medical care. If parents' income is limited to Social Security, or if they deplete their resources, adult children may serve as their parents' safety net at some point during their last years, either by providing care themselves or by paying for needed care and other expenses (Willis 1995).

Long-term care costs are a special worry for older Americans (see Poliaszek 1991). Despite estimates that about 40 percent of those over age 65 will need some type of long-term care, fewer than one-third have provided for this possibility (Willis 1995). Parents and their children may evaluate whether a long-term care policy is cost-effective or consider other ways of financing such care. Policies are expensive, especially at older ages.

Living Arrangements

An AARP survey found that 84 percent of Americans 55 years and over wanted to stay in their own home. However, 54 percent of older Americans had not made plans to ensure that they will have the future housing arrangements they want (Alberts 1995, 56). When aging relatives are unable to manage alone in their own home, they and their adult children will have to explore alternative living arrangements. If adult children live in another part of the country, decisions become more complicated. It is not easy for adult children who live nearby, either. They may resent the fact that they must spend so much time on caregiving because their siblings live far away. They also may be uncomfortable taking responsibility for decisions.

A crisis is reached for many older women and men when they can no longer drive, an event that decreases their independence. In areas without mass transportation, they have to rely on others for mobility. Getting around in a rural or sparsely populated area can be extremely difficult. Some areas do not have taxi services, and many suburbs have no mass transportation. A transportation service may be available for medical appointments, but not for visiting friends, attending social functions or shopping. Not surprisingly, many older persons suffer from depression since this milestone signifies new limits on independence and mobility. Some older persons refuse to accept that they can no longer safely drive and may defy the limitation by continuing to do so, causing concern for their relatives.

Experts advise that elderly relatives always be included in decisions (Zal 1992, 196-197). If changes in living arrangements are forced on parents, they may refuse to move or be so unhappy in their new surroundings that another change is necessary. The disruption in their lives is multiplied and their adjustment becomes even more difficult.

Possible options are for elderly relatives to remain in their own homes with needed support and environmental modifications, to live with relatives or in a residential setting with services. Each alternative has advantages and disadvantages, and a perfect solution may not be possible. Staying at home limits the disorientation that aging individuals may experience in a new setting, but it may raise concerns about their personal safety and nutrition. Community services and support for seniors living at home or with relatives include adult day care, Meals on Wheels, nursing services, transportation, home or health care. A home also may need modifications for convenience and safety.

Residential care facilities range from basically independent apartment living to assisted-living arrangements to nursing homes with several levels of medical care (Zal 1992, 196-197; Wilcox 1996). Some apartment complexes allow residents to be independent but also provide services like housekeeping and meals (Levy 1991; Friedan 1993). Meals may be included, or residents may pay only for meals eaten in the dining room. Other arrangements offer a home-like atmosphere for residents who have their own rooms while meals, housekeeping and laundry services are provided by staff.

Various congregate housing arrangements are possible for older individuals who do not want to live alone but do not need an assisted-living facility (see Levitin 1994, 411-433). Although not available in all areas, communal arrangements may be an economical arrangement for a parent who wants to live with congenial people. Some individuals make arrangements with friends to share housing. Friedan (1993) describes arrangements in which unrelated aging adults live together in a house. Those in good health can manage with a minimum of support.

Aging parents with serious medical problems may need nursing home care. Although such arrangements meet their safety and physical care needs, they have drawbacks as well. If a parent's condition just borders on needing this level of care, the loss of independence and the institutional setting may make adjustment difficult. They also may deteriorate in the institutional setting. The decision is a wrenching one for both parents and children.

Financial considerations play an important role in the decision-making. So will the kinds of care paid for by government programs and health insurance plans. Since regulations and coverage change frequently in these areas, check with authorities and experts in the field on the current status. Families with limited resources may opt for nursing home care if it will paid for by Medicaid, even though other options might be preferable. Since long-term home help is expensive, some families may not be able to afford this choice.

Taking a parent into the home is rare, except for short periods before death or institutionalization. Slightly more than one million Americans who are 65 years or older live with their adult children. In the black community, with a tradition of extended families sharing resources and assisting each other, older relatives frequently are cared for by kin. These kinship arrangements are not necessarily based on blood relationships. Whether extended family households will be as prevalent in the future is uncertain. Dilworth-Anderson (1993, 60-62) suggests that black families may find caring for others more difficult, given factors such as widespread unemployment and increased numbers of single-parent households. Aging blacks who are living longer may be especially affected, since younger relatives may not be able to care for them. Both kinkeepers and caregivers may need support if the arrangement is to continue.

Retrospective questions in a study by Bumpass and Aquilino (1995, 27) revealed that about 25 percent of the sample by late midlife had a parent or a parent-in-law living with them. Few differences existed by race, but the phenomenon was inversely related to education, perhaps because low-income families lacked the financial resources for other types of care.

The very old are more likely to live with adult children (Shapiro 1994, 2). Other options may be possible when children want their parents to live nearby. Granny apartments are one way for parents to remain independent but live with their children. In a newer approach, called Elder Cottage Housing Opportunity (ECHO), children build a temporary structure on their property for parents (AARP 1991, 19; OWL 1993). Zoning and other requirements concerning the feasibility of this option need to be checked out with the authorities before construction is begun.

Problems may arise in intergenerational households that stem from differing views on household management, unresolved conflicts from childhood or clashes between generations on childrearing approaches (Zal 1992, 198). Personality clashes or behavior changes relating to the older person's dementia or Alzheimer's may make life difficult for others in the household. If the parent has a degenerative disease, caregiving needs and stress will increase and may make home care impossible.

On the other hand, such arrangements can work out well when parents are in good health and reciprocity is involved. A parent's help with household tasks or child care can make life easier for working mothers or shared expenses may raise everyone's standard of living (Levy 1991).

Practical Suggestions

Providing or Arranging for Care

More and more adults in their middle years provide care as older relatives live longer. Data from the National Survey of Families and Households (NSFH) show that 7.5 percent of working-age adults were caring for a parent in 1987 and 15 percent were caring for "a parent, spouse, or other adult" (McLanahan and Monson 1990). Women were most likely to be caregivers, with 20 percent of women between the ages of 35 and 65 providing care; two-thirds of these were caring for adults aged 65 or over.

The most difficult situation may be when the older person is in relatively good health but needs a little help daily. The problem may be short-term memory loss or increased frailty that raise fears about falling or other injuries. Facilities providing care seem to be geared to the extremes, either for older persons who are completely independent or for those who need considerable care. Hiring someone to provide assistance in the home several hours daily may be the best arrangement, but it is expensive and works only with reliable caregivers (see AARP 1989; Razzi 1996). Another option is for family members to volunteer to provide care.

When parents can no longer manage independently, the shift in parent-adult child relationships can be difficult for all family members. Characterizing the situation as "role reversal" is inaccurate. Parents are still parents, even when they rely on others for assistance. As Vivian E. Greenberg (quoted in Shapiro 1994, 2) comments: "Our parents never become our children. If we do too much, we take away their autonomy." Loss of independence is frightening to aging individuals, whether it involves giving up driving or accepting help with bathing and getting dressed. The possibility of being helpless in a nursing home or hospital haunts almost all Americans, regardless of their age.

If a parent chooses to stay at home, the living space may have to be modified to eliminate hazards and to provide supports for the older person. Family Enterprises in Milwaukee offers an Elder Safety Kit. The Older Women's League (OWL) and AARP are among the organizations that also offer helpful materials. Emergency devices either can be worn by older persons and those with health problems, or they can be installed in their homes so that they can signal for emergency assistance (Alberts 1995, 57; Family Service America 1990). Since these devices rely on the older person's ability to signal for help, they may be ineffective in some crisis situations. They also may require that a relative or other designated person be available to respond to an emergency. However, they can give older persons and their relatives some peace of mind.

Adult children often assume responsibility for providing care themselves. Many add these daily or weekly caregiving chores to their schedules. Some women spend many hours daily caring for an incapacitated or bedridden relative, which makes for a very long work day. Women usually assume these tasks for their own parents and often for their husbands' parents as well.

Older persons may need assistance in a variety of areas, depending on their conditions. Many need help with daily living and housekeeping chores or assistance with medications or mobility. Others need assistance with grocery shopping, laundry, transportation and going to medical appointments.

Tips for Caregivers

Learning to Cope

Numerous books and articles offer advice on how to cope with aging parents--see, for example, Alberts 1995, Carter and Golant 1995, Horne 1985, Levy 1991, Mall 1990, Smith 1992. However, experience taught me that no amount of reading about elder care and aging parents prepares an individual for the pain experienced when an older person becomes dependent on others. The younger person may find this transition traumatic as well. The situation is especially difficult if they have to be the advocates for changing living arrangements. They may be accused of being cruel, thoughtless or selfish. Yet when medical personnel advise that an older person can no longer live alone, changes must be made. Moreover, those who spend the most time with the individual may make the most accurate assessment of their needs. The situation may come as a surprise for out-of-town relatives, since the individual may function adequately during their visits and they do not see the daily ups-and-downs in the person's behavior and experiences.

Dealing with strong or difficult personalities can make a tough situation worse. Older individuals who see their independence and control slipping away may want to retain whatever control they can, magnifying small decisions into make-or-break battles. Rosalynn Carter (1994) wrote about the family's unsuccessful attempts to convince her determined mother-in-law to have help during her last illness and how they dealt with the situation. Children may have to let their parents make their own decisions, even when they disagree with them. For their part, some parents complain that their children undermine their independence and do not let them make decisions; they begin to treat them as though they were the children.

It often is difficult to convince parents to move out of familiar surroundings for a less comfortable arrangement, especially if they insist that they can manage. Some social workers recommend transferring a person whose health is an issue directly from the hospital to a new setting rather than having them go home first. It seems unfair, but experience seems to show that their adjustment is easier. Individuals who return home first insist that they can manage and may refuse to move to a new place. Of course, whenever possible, the older person should participate by visiting the best facilities and making a choice.

Making New Living Arrangements

The search for an acceptable alternative will depend largely on the options available in the community, as well as the financial resources of the older person and other family members who might contribute to the costs. Some suggestions for approaching the task are:

- Get in touch with the local regional group on aging (the exact name depends on the community) for an orientation to what is available in independent and assisted-living facilities. Those offering levels of care, from minimal assistance to full nursing care, may be preferable if your parent's condition is likely to deteriorate so that they will not have to face several disruptive moves.
- Use available community resources, employee assistance programs at work, and check with friends and colleagues for ideas and recommendations.
- Attend informational meetings, fairs, etc., for older persons. Many organizations offer free brochures and other information.
- Send for information from national organizations concerned with living arrangements for the elderly for information on how to assess facilities.
- Determine how facilities being considered are rated by county, state, national or other agencies providing certification, doing inspections and so on. The rating agency may differ according to the area of the country.
- It is important to get an assessment from a physician and geriatric social worker about your parent's level of functioning and areas where help is needed since the appropriate type of facility will be determined by this information. Also find out what your parent will consider and which arrangements would be most acceptable. Bear in mind, though, that people change their minds, and your parent may decide on something different from what was expected.
- Visit a number of facilities in the community, perhaps ranging from large apartment complexes for seniors to smaller group homes. Either do this in the company of your parent or narrow the possibilities down and visit these together to avoid too much running around, disappointments and confusion.

Some steps to take in assessing an assisted-living residence include:

- Check references and talk to current or former residents about the home or facility.
- Get information on the number and qualifications of staff. What is the ratio of staff to residents during the day? How many staff members are there at night? How do staff and residents relate to each other?
- Find out what level of health care is available. Is a nurse available at all times? Is a doctor on premises or on call 24 hours?
- Check out the status of safety and other inspections.
- Are other residents functioning at about the same level as your relative? You don't want to place your alert parent in a facility with a preponderance of Alzheimer's patients. Do other residents seem satisfied with the setting?
- Does the facility belong to any associations of caregiving organizations?
- How does the home rate in terms of cleanliness and type of furnishings? Can a resident bring furniture and other items from home?
- Are there planned activities and outings? How frequent are they?
- What services are provided? Meals? Personal care assistance? Laundry? Medication? Special diets?
- Is the food nourishing and well-prepared? Can a resident's dietary restrictions and preferences be accommodated? I visited a small group home whose manager did not seem familiar with a diabetic diet. It seems hard to believe, since so many older persons control their blood sugar through oral medication and diet.

The important question is how your relative reacted to the surroundings, the staff and the other residents. Some older persons may prefer a smaller setting to a larger, more impersonal institutional facility with more services and activities. For example, the large dining room in one highly rated facility that I visited with my aunt intimidated her. She preferred a much smaller group home. In some areas, the choices may be limited and no arrangement is ideal. You and your parent may have to decide what's most important and settle for less than desired accommodations.

If a nursing home is indicated by the older person's condition, intensive investigation of possible places is essential. This procedure entails checking with licensing authorities, determining whether complaints have been filed, and visiting the facility several times. Check not only that it is certified, but also whether it belongs to national organizations. It is a good idea to visit a nursing home unannounced to see the place under those circumstances. The staff's policies concerning use of restraints and medication for patients is another important concern for families. Other aspects of the facility's services, staff and attitudes toward individuals to review are similar to those discussed above for assisted-living facilities. Many organizations offer advice and checklists to assist you in assessing nursing homes; see, for example, Carter and Golant 1994, 183-

189; Health and Human Services 1994; Levine 1995; Smith 1992; Family Service America; and an evaluation form from Children of Aging Parents (CAPS).

The elder person should play an active role in the decision-making, even though the resulting arrangement may not seem the best one from the children's or professionals' point of view. Whether or not the decision is viable will become evident. It may take time to develop a workable solution, with negotiations and adaptations required by all involved. Arrangements cannot be forced on the parent or other older relative who considers them unacceptable.

Home Care Advice

If the decision is that your parent will stay at home, with household or health care assistance, some practical tips for arranging and supervising care include:

- Consider a geriatric care manager if you live far away and can afford the cost.
- Look into nurse registries, home health agencies and similar sources to find the required personnel. These might include nurses, therapists, homemaker services, home health or personal care aides, and so on.
- Verify that a home care services agency is licensed and accredited.
- Make sure that the people you hire to provide care are honest and reliable. Check out individuals with agencies and contact former employers for recommendations. Home health aides require little or no special training, although many are experienced practical nurses. Does the agency provide training? Sometimes, too, an aide's personality, willingness to do the job, and relationship with the older person are more important than specialized training if care needs are not complicated. If they are good at their job and establish a rapport with the older person, do not be surprised if your parent seems more interested and involved with them than with you. Remember that they spend many hours together and if you live out of town you visit only for short periods. Be happy that your parent has congenial companionship, rather than being jealous about this new relationship.
- Always try to have a few extra caregivers available and willing to fill in if needed, especially for 24-hour care. Anyone who has relied on outside help knows that they will have emergencies, whether it be illness, family responsibilities or car trouble. Have a "Plan B" to fall back on at all times.
- Use available local resources to make caregiving easier and to improve the quality of life of the older individual. These services include Meals on Wheels, Visiting Nurse Service, home health aides, adult day care and medical transportation services.

Those who have arranged home care often have horror stories about unreliable, dishonest, careless or disinterested workers. One of my experiences involves an elderly relative discharged from the hospital after a heart attack with an aide supplied by the hospital to assist her. When she went to her bank several weeks later, she found that the aide had stolen a check and withdrawn all the money from her account. (She got her money back because the bank was liable.) Don't be discouraged, though, because other members of my family in several geographic areas have had excellent home care experiences. The women hired went beyond the expected in providing care and were reliable in maintaining their schedules, even putting in extra hours when needed. It may take some trial and error before reliable arrangements are established, but be persistent.

If you have primary responsibility for care, experts recommend that an overriding task is to keep yourself healthy and able to bear the strain. If you become ill, then the whole caregiving setup is imperiled. There is even a "Caregivers' Bill of Rights" (Horne 1985) to remind you to think of yourself. Some specific suggestions include:

- Make sure that you have a backup plan in case something happens and you cannot be there.
- Make time for yourself, even if this means hiring outside help for a few hours weekly.
- Plan activities that you enjoy with friends and family, and use stress management techniques. Also seek out support groups. Genovese (1984b) has described how self-help groups meet family needs, especially when formal programs do not exist. These groups provide helpful suggestions about caregiving, negotiating the bureaucratic maze, and identifying sources of help. You can learn what works and what does not, rather than finding out by trial and error; see Carter and Golant (1994), Smith (1992), Norris (1988) and other books on support groups. Children of Aging Parents (CAPS) has a manual for starting such a group if there isn't one in your area.
- Enlist other family members to contribute time, money or whatever they can.

Regardless of how devoted a caregiver is, she or he may experience a range of emotions, from grief and sadness to anger, guilt, resentment and fear (Carter and Golant 1994, 76-87; Shapiro 1991, 155-85; Smith 1992, 89-90; Zal 1992, 204-208). Caregivers often think that they are not doing enough, even when they are exhausted by their demanding schedules (Greenberg 1989). In fact, family members may continue to provide home care when aging relatives really need skilled nursing care. Experts advise adult children or other relatives not to make promises to the older person that they may not be able to keep, especially the promise that they will never let them go to a nursing home since that step may be unavoidable at some future time.

Managing care from afar may involve a good deal of administrative work, especially to ensure that help is in place when required, which is hard to do from miles away. It might be possible to assign one paid caregiver the responsibility for managing the schedule. Another option is to hire a geriatric care manager. Arranging payment for caregivers is a logistical issue, since the mail can be unreliable. If the older person needs assistance during the night, then a live-in caregiver can eliminate scheduling problems.

Integrating Caregiving with Work

The high labor force participation of mid-life women, who are the primary providers or managers of care to aging relatives, makes this responsibility more difficult than ever. Women may experience high stress levels from caregiving in addition to working full time, managing a household and perhaps raising children.

Employers have responded to workers who are juggling work and childrearing responsibilities by offering programs and services, but they have been much slower to assist those with elder care responsibilities. A small number of companies have pioneered in this area. Perhaps surprisingly, government has been even slower than the private sector to introduce programs and policies in this area.

One reason for these different responses is the greater prevalence and visibility of child care issues among workers. Another reason stems from employees' reluctance to call attention to their elder care responsibilities. Workers may fear that their performance ratings will be affected or that they will be considered not committed to their jobs. Workers are particularly hesitant to use elder care responsibilities as a reason for being late or for taking time off.

A frequent employee benefit is the dependent care assistance program (DCAP). This program allows employees to set aside pretax dollars for dependent care costs, whether for children or adults. Since the money not used by the end of the year is forfeited, some employees are reluctant to participate (AARP *Working Age* 1995, 4-5).

Employers are experimenting with a variety of elder care programs and services with varying success. Employees' use of resource and referral services in some companies has been low and success mixed. Workers who use this service consider it a big time-saver (Lawlor 1995). On the other hand, flextime is very popular, perhaps because it benefits those with child care *or* parent care responsibilities.

Some companies have expanded elder care offerings to include direct services. For example, a "resource and referral" service may include an assessment of an older person's status and needs by a health services agency and recommendations for needed services. Adult day care centers have had mixed success, and employers in some communities dropped respite care programs because older persons did not want strangers in their home.

Projects of the American Business Collaborative for Quality Dependent Care, whose members include AT&T, IBM, Xerox and GTE, have been well-received. Programs are tailored to workers' needs in a specific community. For example, an emergency backup care program for Xerox employees pays approximately two-thirds of a substitute caregiver's salary when a child or parent is sick or a regular caregiver is unable to work. After negotiations with two unions, AT&T set up a family care development fund whose programs include national expansion of Meals on Wheels, as well as adult day care centers, caregiver support groups and respite care to allow caregivers a break (Lawlor 1995).

Employer interest in how much elder care costs them is growing. A recent study by the Washington Business Group on Health (Coberly and Hunt 1995) tried to quantify these costs to an unidentified manufacturer with a work force of almost 87,000. An estimated 2 percent of employees were providing personal care to older relatives--spouses, parents, parents-in-law and grandparents. This estimate is low since it includes only personal care. Furthermore, long-distance care costs and other assistance such as financial management, administering medication, cooking or transportation were excluded. Moreover, three-quarters of the company's work force, and 84 percent of those between the ages of 50 and 64 were men, but most elder care is provided by women.

The total cost to the employer was an estimated $5.5 million. However, studies estimate that as many as 12 percent of workers provide care to older relatives. Using that figure, employer costs could be as high as $33 million.

Replacement costs for employees who quit their jobs, absenteeism, interruptions during the work day and elder care crises were included in the estimate. Supervision, health and mental health costs also were estimated. Additional costs that could not be quantified were leaves of absence, reduced work schedules or job changes, impact on other employees and human capital issues such as declined promotions, transfers, missed meetings or trips, and passed-up chances for continued education (Coberly and Hunt 1995, 6-12). Costs to *employees* were not considered in detail. It is not clear how this kind of assessment will affect employers. Will it spur them to offer more programs--or make them more interested in monitoring employees with elder care responsibilities? Employees may become even more reluctant to discuss their responsibilities for elder care.

More companies can be expected to focus on elder care issues with baby boomers now turning 50. Managers facing these concerns in their own lives may be more sympathetic to employees' concerns and pressures. In a Families and Work Institute study (Galinsky et al. 1993), 18 percent of employees surveyed expected to be involved in elder care in the near future; the figure rose to more than 25 percent for those 50 years or older. The productivity costs for personal caregivers, figured as 18 percent of the work force, would be more than $17 billion--an astounding figure.

POLICY ISSUES: WHO CARES FOR AND ABOUT THE ELDERLY?

Many policy issues arise with regard to older Americans, especially centering around the economics of aging and the politics and policies of elder care. Proposed public policy changes could have serious potential consequences for older Americans today and in the future. Some of the issues are discussed below.

Also at issue is the distribution of society's resources to benefit citizens. Government programs have played a major role in decreasing poverty among older Americans during the past decades. Now young people are asking whether they will receive the same benefits in their later years as their parents and grandparents do. This issue is considered in chapter 6.

Adult children who already are struggling to help with the cost of their parents' care, or providing the care themselves, may be expected to do more (Winik 1995). An article by Crowley and Glasheen (1996) in the AARP *Bulletin*, aptly titled "Should Kids Pay For Mom?" discussed problems for adult children faced with enormous costs for elder care. It obviously received considerable attention, since the April 1996 *Bulletin* contained a number of reader's reactions.

The article discussed lawmakers' proposals that children of the elderly be required to assume some of the financial cost for their care (see Crowley and Glasheen 1996). One of the most controversial proposals would permit states to recover Medicaid nursing home costs from a beneficiary's estate, bringing adult children's responsibility for their parents to a new level. However, its chances of becoming law seem slim.

Those who work in the area of elder care suggest that a different approach to policy is needed. They propose that programs and policies in the areas of taxation, health benefit plans, employment, and social services adopt a lifespan perspective to ease burdens on caregivers and improve care for Americans of all ages (Marks 1993,16).

In a discussion about working for better conditions, Horne (1985) offers a range of proposals to benefit both those giving and receiving care. A major advance would be to provide financial compensation for family caregivers. They also need assistance so that they can provide care without experiencing burnout. More support groups and respite programs for caregivers and adult day care centers would help families. Government funds for respite care are limited today (Hooyman 1992, 196).

Since older Americans are a diverse group, these differences should be reflected in programs and services. More programs are needed for the low-income elderly, those living alone who are disproportionately women, those who could remain in their homes if needed services were covered by public and private health care plans, and the handicapped. Community alternatives to large nursing homes also would allow older individuals who need support to live as independently as possible in a home-like setting. Services would include congregate meals, housekeeping, and help with daily activities. Currently, when such options are available, they tend to be expensive and limited to those with considerable financial resources.

The Family and Medical Leave Act of 1993, passed during the Clinton administration, helps family members who need to take time from their jobs to care for ill or elderly relatives. It provides 12 weeks of unpaid leave, during which time an employee's job is protected (Longo 1995b, 92). Policies also are needed to protect caregivers' retirement benefits when they take time off. Scandinavian policies could provide a model, but the current political climate makes a move in that direction unlikely (Hooyman 1992,199).

Foster and Brizius (1993, 70-71) suggest that a coalition is needed to press for changes in public policy on caregiving. They recommend that advocates for the care of the young, old and the disabled band together and press for increased funding and programs for *all* caregivers. At present, many groups are competing with each other for available funds.

The discussion earlier in this chapter indicated that some large companies now include elder care benefits as part of their employee packages. Workers with elder care responsibilities could benefit from more information and referral assistance, as well as flexible scheduling opportunities. More widespread benefits for part-time workers also are important. Many workers cannot afford to cut back on their hours because they will lose benefits. Such policies tend to perpetuate inequities for women who are most likely to modify or shorten their work schedules to meet caregiving needs.

Some employers allow workers to use their sick time to meet the care needs of other family members. With this issue, as with other employee requests, companies often prefer to use a informal case-by-case approach rather than making such policies official. In the downsizing and layoff environment of today's corporation, new and costly programs often are unpopular. Moreover, employees who worry about their jobs are not likely to draw attention to their family responsibilities by pushing for elder care benefits (Seccombe 1992, 174-175).

The issue of combining work and elder care, however, will not go away. As the number of aging baby boomers with elder care responsibilities grows, this generation may become advocates for new and improved programs. They also may lead the way in gaining greater acceptance of elder care as an important focus for mid-life adults and increasing work place flexibility for employees who assume such duties.

CHAPTER 5

Women at Midlife: In Their Prime?

INTRODUCTION

Women at midlife face special planning issues because they live longer than men and face possible economic insecurity in later life. A variety of economic and social factors over their lifetime can adversely affect women's status in late life: discrimination, years out of the labor force for homemaking and child care, unequal pay and benefits, limited opportunities for job training or retraining, part-time and contingent work with no benefits, and divorce or early widowhood (Pifer 1993, 245).

Although the phrase "alone at last" is often used to refer to mid-life couples who have entered the "empty nest" phase of marriage, it has special meaning for women who tend to be "alone at the last"; they are likely to be alone during their last years, regardless of whether they are widowed, divorced or never married. In 1988 there were 11.2 million widows, but only 2.3 million widowers in the United States, counting only those not in nursing homes or other institutions. Almost one-half of the women aged 65 or over were widowed (Saluter 1989, 4-5).

Women also spend more years in widowhood, averaging 15.3 years, compared to only 8.4 years for men. Older African-American women are less likely than older white or Hispanic women to be married and are more likely to be widowed, given black men's higher mortality rates. They also are more likely to be divorced or never married (Taeuber and Allen 1993, 28). In general, more adults are single today compared to 1970, owing largely to postponed marriage or divorce, increasing the likelihood that many will never marry and may be alone in later life. (Saluter 1989, 1).

The aging of the population and increased longevity means that mid-life women today can expect to spend more time as caregivers in later life. They may meet these caregiving demands at the expense of their own economic well-being (and health). Pifer (1993, 252) takes the position that the cost of our society's adjustment to population aging has been borne mainly by women.

Moreover, the situation is not likely to change. As medical advances help those with chronic illnesses to live longer, they will need care either at home or in assisted-living facilities (Pifer 1993, 244). Longer periods of caregiving will increase the stress experienced by mid-life and older women. Health care cost-cutting may place even more onus on family members to provide care, perhaps without home health care services to make their job easier. As women live longer, they themselves are likely to need care and may have fewer relatives to support them. Many will be poor as well. Planning for the future, then, is especially important for women.

ECONOMIC SECURITY AT MIDLIFE AND BEYOND

Although retirement is probably the farthest thing from a young woman's mind when she starts her first job, financial advisors recommend that she begin planning for the future as early as possible. Housing, car payments, children's education, and other expenditures seem more important and immediate to a young worker. However, if a woman waits until midlife to start saving, she will find it difficult to put aside enough for later life. Unless they have accumulated sufficient resources by their late 50s or 60s, many women will not be able to retire. They even may find themselves working at minimum-wage jobs just to survive, since their Social Security payments may not keep them above the poverty level.

Social scientists have pointed out the diverse economic circumstances of both couples and women in their later years. Articles by Allen, Malveaux, Taeuber and Allen and other contributors to *Women on the Front Lines* (Allen and Pifer 1993) focus on the economic, health and social circumstances of women in our aging society. On the one hand, some couples enjoy sizable pensions, investments and homes with greatly appreciated values. Their lifestyle in retirement is comparable to when one or both worked. Many of these women will continue to live comfortably after their spouse dies. Widows control considerable wealth in this country.

In contrast, single women with a lifetime of low-paying jobs may have to rely on Social Security in retirement, perhaps supplemented by a small pension. Widowed or divorced women who never worked or had part-time or minimum-wage jobs may be poor in the last decades of life. Other women will be poor because they left the labor force or worked at part-time jobs so that they could care for a parent, spouse or other relative.

Today's older women may have few assets for work-related reasons: lower-paying jobs, often in female-dominated occupations; part-time and contingent jobs; unequal pay; and time out of the labor force for child and elder care responsibilities. Many elderly widows become poor because their income shrinks after their spouse dies. They may lose all or part of his pension income. In some instances, his last illness will have used up most of their assets, especially if he required nursing home care. Spousal impoverishment is an unwelcome possibility for many women in late life (Stone 1989; Davis et al. 1990).

Working at Midlife

Many women approaching midlife today have more economic advantages and resources than their mothers did at their age, owing to their higher educational levels and better-paying jobs. However, women know that a higher education does not necessarily translate into higher salaries and that the pay gap between men and women has not disappeared. A *Working Woman* (1995) survey suggests that the gap has narrowed to 74 percent, compared to 59 percent in the late 1960s or 1970s. (However, some experts question this estimate because the survey was not representative of all women in the work force.)

The narrowing gap is not necessarily a cause for celebration, because it results partly from men's falling wages: "This is not exactly what we meant when we said we wanted to catch up with men, that their wages should fall in real terms" (Hartmann 1995, 3). The Women's Policy Research (IWPR) calculates that about three-fifths of women's progress is attributable to men's falling wages.

In the future, women who enter the labor force early and work continuously until retirement age will have larger Social Security benefits in their own right, as well as more chances for traditional pensions and 401(k) plans. With continuous labor force participation and perhaps portable pensions, their assets can grow appreciably by retirement. Yet economic security still may be beyond the reach of women earning the minimum wage or a little more.

Ethnic background is an important determinant of women's economic status at midlife. Despite the progress many minority women have made in educational attainment and employment, they still earn less than white women and men. Those trapped in low-paying jobs, often without health care or pension benefits, constantly struggle to raise their incomes above the poverty level and to achieve a measure of economic security.

Some low-income women may improve their economic well-being by working at nontraditional blue-collar jobs with better salaries and benefits than many secretarial and clerical jobs. Additionally, these occupations are likely to be organized, another advantage since research indicates that women's wages tend to increase more than men's do with union membership (Hartmann 1995, 10).

Minority women's work experience affects their later life status in other ways as well. As Malveaux (1993) notes, minority women are more likely than white women to work "off the books," so that they may lack both a pension and Social Security benefits. Household workers, whose employers did not pay the requisite taxes on their wages, are not even eligible for Social Security benefits based on those earnings. Poverty for older women of color, especially black women, stems more from past work experience than from marital status. Therefore, minority women's later-life economic status will be affected by such factors as continuous work histories, occupational and educational backgrounds, family responsibilities, and health (Malveaux 1993,187).

Minority women also will make up a growing proportion of the 65-and-over population in the future and will constitute more of the "oldest old." By 2030, there will be 4.4 million black women aged 65 and over. If current trends continue, 1.7 million of them would be poor and another .9 million would be near the poverty level (Malveaux 1993, 175).

To make ends meet, women are more likely than men to hold more than one job, often because they work at minimum-wage jobs or as contingent workers. They are estimated to hold about 60 to 65 percent of the less-desirable jobs.

Both women and men worry about job security. They may be victims of corporate "downsizing" and lose pension benefits as well as current income. If they are the last hired, women may be the first to be let go in a round of job cuts. Consequently, a sizable proportion of younger women still may rely primarily on Social Security payments in their later years, despite years of labor force participation.

On the other hand, women are making inroads into better-paying jobs; increasing numbers are in professional and managerial jobs, and more also are becoming entrepreneurs. Self-employment has tripled since 1970 (Hartmann 1995, 12). Some women choose this option to make it easier to combine work with family responsibilities. Other women have begun businesses after bumping up against the "glass ceiling" and finding advancement blocked in large organizations [see, for example, U.S. Merit Systems Protection Board (1992) on the glass ceiling in government]. These women have the potential for high incomes, increasing their ability to accumulate assets and plan for a secure retirement. However, they also have a greater need to save for retirement if they have no pension plan.

This discussion underscores why financial planning is so important for women. Yet despite considerable work experience and earning capacity, some women still are uncomfortable about managing their assets or making joint financial decisions with their spouses.

Managing Finances and Planning for Retirement

A woman's pension nest egg and Social Security payments will be important in the timing of retirement. Marital status also will influence her retirement decision. If she is married, the decision will be a joint one, as discussed in chapter 2. A study by Morgan (1992) found that marital status was a factor in decisions about *when* and *whether* to retire. Formerly married women planned to retire about two years later than their married counterparts did. Not surprisingly, married women expected to have more sources of post-retirement income than did those without spouses. Retaining health care benefits also may play an important role in a woman's decision to continue working.

Given their longevity and the possibility of having only their own resources in later life, young women should start learning to manage their money when they begin to work. Learning early is also good preparation for managing money in retirement. If they become widowed or divorced and their spouse made all of the financial decisions, they may have no idea how to proceed. As an account executive with a brokerage firm, I learned that some older women have never written a check or balanced a checkbook. If widowed suddenly, they would be unprepared to make important and perhaps irrevocable financial decisions. They may not know what their joint assets are, how much income they have, or where it comes from. They may not even have such basic facts as how much their husband earned or what pension benefits they receive on his death.

At this difficult time, they are especially vulnerable to unscrupulous financial salespeople who may steer them to risky investments or give them investment advice based on the commissions they will make. Women often have been easy targets for brokers who make risky investments for them, while assuring them that they are conservative and can't lose money. Recently widowed women without investment experience may be especially subject to pressure to sign trading power over their account to a stockbroker or financial advisor. Some women have regretted hasty financial decisions made after a spouse's death when they were in mourning.

Powers (1996, F11) describes the financial pitfalls and mistakes she made in an article entitled "A Widow's Walk on the Wild Side." Others may seek help with decision-making from their spouse's employers who may not be prepared to offer such support to deceased employees' families. Other companies have set up special services to help survivors. Survivors also may face volumes of paperwork to determine decisions to be made about health insurance, life insurance, pensions and 401(k) plans, and Social Security payments (see White 1995; Schultz 1994, C1).

On the other hand, many women are extremely competent in financial matters. They manage their own and their family's finances, invest regularly, and are comfortable making investment decisions. Others assume responsibility for their own current finances, but may not make long-range financial plans for retirement. A lack of confidence in their own judgment may lead women to avoid what they consider "risky" investments. Even women with successful careers may be nervous about investing or losing money.

Willis's (1996b) list of money management mistakes typically made by women includes being too conservative because they fear the wrong risk--of losing money in a volatile stock market rather than of inflation eroding the value of their savings. They also tend to assume that their current financial status is permanent or to wait for the right time to save, rather than starting right away with small amounts.

Mid-life women today tend to have smaller pension benefits for work-related reasons already discussed. Defined contribution plans, which depend on employee contributions, may mean that fewer women will be eligible for them or that their pensions will be smaller because they cannot afford to save money regularly. Single parents supporting families on modest salaries will not be able to contribute much, but they still should put aside whatever they can on a regular basis. The total amount saved by retirement also will depend on how the money was invested over time and whether any funds were withdrawn from the plan before retirement. It is relatively easy for employees to tap into such plans for emergencies and the money may not be replaced.

Therefore, all women need to learn to manage their money and make financial plans, regardless of their age, marital status, occupation or income level. Singles especially need to plan because their incomes tend to be less than a married couple's and they may have only one income at retirement (see Longo 1996).

Starting to Plan

Take Control of Your Finances

The first steps in planning for economic security are often the hardest. Hannon (1995, 22) offers five rules to help women reach their financial goals: (1) "Make Saving for Retirement Your Top Financial Priority"; (2) "If You're Married, Manage Your Finances As If You Are Going to Be Alone One Day"; (3) "Know and Protect What's Rightfully Yours"; (4) "Force yourself to take risks with your money"; and (5) "Consider the financial implications of career moves." She also advises them to take into account the possibility that they may be alone at some point(s) during adulthood.

The first task is to figure out your expenses, what you will need to live on, and how much you have to save and invest to meet your goal. If married, figure out your own assets and liabilities, independent of your spouse's, as well as your joint status (see chapter 2 for information). Decide how much you can save on a regular basis and stick to putting that amount of money away. If you lack the discipline, you can have funds automatically withdrawn from your paycheck and deposited in a savings or investment account.

Take advantage of employer offers to match your contributions to a retirement plan. Try to make other investments as well, including building a portfolio of stocks or mutual funds and contributing to an IRA, if neither you nor your spouse has a retirement plan. If you are self-employed, retirement planning should not be ignored, even though your energies are directed mainly to keeping your business afloat. Setting up a SEP/IRA or Keogh plan is an excellent move. Also decide whether to contribute to a nondeductible Individual Retirement Account (IRA).

Some specific financial planning steps to consider include the following:

Plan Ahead for Unexpected Emergencies

Various crises can threaten your own and your family's financial security. These unexpected disasters include layoffs, disability, death or divorce. It is essential for a single parent to protect against hard times. De Yoe (1995) suggests doing the following: set up an emergency fund, take out disability protection, assess your life insurance needs, and have an umbrella insurance policy. This advice is equally important for men.

Experts recommend that your rainy day savings should amount to three to six months of living expenses, depending on your circumstances. You can never go wrong setting aside more funds than you expect to need. You hope never to tap into the money, but it can be a lifesaver in an emergency. If untouched, the amount will make a nice addition to your retirement nest egg. Since the money should be readily available, a money market fund or short-term certificate of deposit (CD) is a good place for it.

Another potential lifesaver can be a credit card. This advice may seem strange since many credit-card users run up too much debt and pay astounding amounts in interest charges. On a recent television program, a divorced single parent told how she ran up $40,000 in credit-card debt and had to declare bankruptcy. However, these cards can be an essential tool in helping individuals and families to survive a financial crisis or emergency like an unexpected layoff or medical costs.

Many people don't think about disability insurance until they are unable to work for medical reasons and it is too late. Both men and women workers should have this protection, whether single or married. An insurance company study found that "only 18% of its policy holders who own individual disability-insurance policies are working women, even though 55% of all women contribute at least half of their families' income" (De Yoe 1995, 27). Women also file more claims than men do. Many employers offer such coverage, but group plans may not replace a high enough proportion of lost income. You might want to consider whether to buy an expensive supplemental policy as well.

Review your insurance coverage to decide whether it is adequate, whether you need life insurance, and what amount makes sense. If you are single with no children, you may not need any; if you are a single parent, you do. Since health care costs can drain the assets of any family, consider whether to increase health coverage at midlife when medical costs may rise. As you approach retirement age, consider whether to buy Medigap insurance to cover deductibles for hospital stays, home health care and other expenses (Hannon 1995, 24). New tax breaks for long-term care insurance may make such policies more popular. An umbrella liability protection policy can be beneficial as well. Because lawsuits are so common, it can protect your own and your family's assets in case you are sued (De Yoe 1995, 82).

Take Action to Protect Your Interests

Being financially knowledgeable makes sense for women today, whether they are single or married. If married, learn everything you can about your joint assets and liabilities. Most women know that they should establish credit in their own name, and many have their own savings and investment accounts. They may be less aware of their liability for a spouse's debt or for a joint income-tax return. White (1995) covers some implications of marriage, divorce, retirement, estates and other topics for married women.

A few words of warning. If you co-sign a loan agreement, mortgage or other type of debt jointly with your spouse, read the documents carefully and understand what you are agreeing to. If you are unsure about the implications, get a professional to interpret the legal jargon and explain your liability. Also be aware of your liability when you sign a joint return, as numerous women were dismayed to learn after the fact. (Of course, liability goes both ways; husbands may be responsible for debts of their spouses as well.) Legislation has been proposed to change this situation, given the hardships faced by spouses saddled with large tax bills because of their partners' actions.

If you and your spouse are negotiating a divorce, be sure that the settlement is fair and includes part of your ex-spouse's retirement benefits earned during the marriage. Legal advice can help you get an equitable settlement. To share in his pension, you must get a Qualified Domestic Relations Order (QDRO), a court order or court-approved agreement between the parties for sharing the pension according to the Employee Retirement Income Security Act (ERISA). Furthermore, if you were married for ten or more years and do not remarry, at 62 years of age you will qualify for Social Security benefits based on your ex-spouse's earnings, regardless of whether he has remarried or still is working and not receiving benefits (Older Women's League 1995).

Prenuptial agreements are common today, and not just for the wealthy. To some, the step seems unromantic; to others, it looks like good common sense. If you are remarrying and have children from a previous marriage, a prenuptial agreement can ensure that your children will inherit your estate. Your intended spouse may insist on such a step if he has children from a previous marriage.

Marriage for older persons today has important financial consequences. After some couples figure out what they would lose in income and benefits, they decide to live together without marriage. Remarriage also can eliminate the one-time capital gains tax benefit on the sale of one partner's house if the other has already taken theirs. An accountant can advise on how to handle this issue and whether individual tax returns are indicated. Other couples may find that a divorce is the only way for an ill spouse to receive costly medical or nursing care without impoverishing the other--another example of how policies affect Americans' lives.

Learn About Financial Planning and Investing

To make yourself more confident about making basic investment decisions and planning your future, read basic books, magazines and newspapers. Attend free seminars to get information, but be wary about committing yourself to an investment without further analysis. You may want to ask knowledgeable friends or acquaintances for advice, but make your own decisions. Their priorities, income and resources may differ significantly from yours, so that their investment choices may be inappropriate for you. If you are reluctant to invest on your own, consider joining an investment club. Many women-only clubs have been very successful, as exemplified by the Beardstown Ladies (1994).

Some suggested resources. AARP has published a number of helpful guides and workbooks, including: *A Primer on Financial Management for Midlife and Older Women* (1988); *Tomorrow's Choices: Preparing Now for Future Legal, Financial and Health Care Decisions* (1992b); *Focus Your Future: A Woman's Guide to Retirement Planning* (1991); and *A Woman's Guide to Pension Rights* (1992a). As noted above, *What Every Woman Should Know About Her Husband's Money* (White 1995) has chapters on prenuptial agreements, divorce, wills, estates and the rights of children.

The Prep Project of the National Center for Women and Retirement Research at Long Island University, Southampton, NY has prepared numerous guides for financial planning, including *Looking Ahead to Your Financial Future* and *Employment and Retirement Issues for Women*. Also see Leonard's *Money and the Mature Woman*.

Books such as Jane Bryant Quinn's *Making the Most of Your Money* and Terry Savage's *New Money Strategies for the 1990s* can be useful, general guides on a range of financial and retirement planning issues and questions. Cheryl Broussard (1995) has written a financial planning book for African-American women. Local libraries will have these or similar books on their shelves. *Kiplinger's, Money, Working Woman, Smart Money*, and *Worth* are just a few magazines with regular features on financial topics.

Information and resources also are readily available from government agencies like the Social Security Administration, Women's Bureau, Department of Labor and private organizations like the Pension Rights Center and the Older Women's League (OWL). See the Bibliography and Appendices for publications from these and other organizations.

SOCIAL ASPECTS OF WOMEN'S LATER YEARS

Issues for women at midlife are social as well as economic. It is a time when they may start to plan for the activities and roles that will occupy them after retirement. The National Center for Women and Retirement Research's *Social and Emotional Issues for Mid-life Women* covers such relevant topics as the maturing woman, transitions, changing family relationships and retirement.

It recognizes that some women are in transition and seeking new roles because their other roles, like "mother," "worker," and perhaps "spouse," are being transformed or ending.

Women alone at midlife may relish their independence or be unsure about what kind of life they want after divorce or widowhood. As more women are in this situation, books and seminars offering advice are increasing. For example, a recent book, *Women Home Alone,* by Sprinkle provides information ranging from advice on how to deal with house repairs to surviving the holidays alone.

Some women may want to concentrate on jobs and careers. If embarking on a new career, they can expect to spend years on the job, perhaps beyond the usual retirement age. Work in later life can provide not only needed income, but also the opportunity for social interaction. However, women in their 50s or older may have difficulty finding a job if their skills are limited or obsolete. See AARP's *Returning to the Job Market* (1992) for some ideas on how to go about identifying opportunities. Displaced homemaker programs for women who are divorced or lack job skills helped women in the 1970s obtain training and become self-sufficient. Such programs have little funding today, and displaced homemaker programs vie with other groups for assistance (Jacobs 1993).

Women approaching midlife have more lifestyle options than earlier generations. If they are not in the labor force, they may be involved in community activities and use their skills for paid or volunteer work after retirement. A study of women's longevity concluded that involvement with clubs or other voluntary organizations was related to a long life (Moen et al. 1994, 643). Women who enjoyed social activities associated with work may maintain friendships with co-workers after retirement. Others may choose to travel, go back to school or devote time to hobbies. Many will enjoy spending time with their grandchildren, and some will become caregivers while the children's parents are at work.

Given their work experience, wide interests and many years of retirement, many will not be content to focus on leisure activities and begin to develop more active roles for themselves, perhaps starting new careers or using their skills in decision-making positions in their communities.

Kinkeepers and Caregivers: Women's Roles at Midlife and Beyond

Friedan (1993) suggests that women age better than men because aging is just one of many transitions in their lives. Over a lifetime they may adjust to: marriage and motherhood; entering and leaving the labor force, perhaps several times during their work careers; an empty nest when children leave home, then perhaps return again; divorce and remarriage; their spouse's and their own retirement; years of providing care to various family members; and widowhood. For an analysis of how women's roles change, see Lopata's (1995) *Circles and Settings.*

One role for women has not changed--that of caregiver. In fact, it is taking up more time. Mid-life women can expect many years ahead as caregivers for parents, parents-in-law and spouse. The strains may be considerable, especially for those with multiple caregiving responsibilities, either simultaneously or one after the other. Women face role overload, too, because these responsibilities are added to already full schedules. The caregiver tips discussed in chapter 4 apply largely to women, since they shoulder the main responsibility for elder care.

In general, women act as "kinkeepers," keeping families together over the life cycle. As Aldous (1995, 111) notes, they are primarily responsible for the "well-documented emotional and instrumental glue that keeps lineages together." They are the ones who maintain contact with relatives and organize get-togethers and reunions (Jacobs 1993). They also are the ones who usually remember birthdays, write letters or E-mail communications to distant family members, and visit or keep in touch with ill relatives.

When parents divorce, an adult daughter often takes the lead in keeping family traditions alive if her mother does not continue this role (Pett et al. 1992, 547-548). She also may assume this responsibility if her mother can no longer take the lead in planning gatherings or maintaining contacts with distant relatives.

Women may become family matriarchs in their later years. Some will act as mentors to young family members or acquaintances. They may share their store of knowledge about the family's roots and experiences, which is especially important in black families, for example, with strong oral history traditions (Jacobs 1993, 203). In four-generation families, they may hand down family stories to a succession of younger family members. As discussed in chapter 3, they may play an even more active role in influencing future generations by raising their grandchildren.

In later years, an older person's involvement with family and friends may decrease as some move away and others die. Their mobility also may limit their ability to visit others or attend gatherings. Women cope with these developments in different ways. Some become resigned to staying home and may become isolated; others are able to arrange for transportation and continue to have a busy social life.

Many will face shrinking social networks and even isolation as they age. More women can expect to live alone in their later years. As Taeuber (1993, 30) notes: "Remarriage is not common among elderly women. In addition, more women (especially black women) are entering their elder years as divorced or never married." Some may outlive not only a spouse, but even an adult child. This experience is difficult for many to bear since it is a loss for which they are unprepared (Lipovenko 1996).

Since many women will be alone in their later years, midlife is a good time to begin a process of redefining relationships and creating new ones. Those who are unmarried or divorced in their middle years may build a support network for the future. Childless women or those not close to their children also may develop a circle of friends and relatives to provide companionship and mutual aid as they age. If they don't take this step, they may find themselves "marginalized as social discards" (Jacobs 1993, 191). Their role as kinkeepers offers one direction for the future. If no family members live nearby, they may establish surrogate family relationships with unrelated individuals. These may be informal or may lead to creating new "families" and households with friends or acquaintances. Even whole families, young and old, make efforts to develop family-like relationships with congenial others, sometimes because their own families are scattered in other parts of the country. They celebrate holidays as a group and get together on a regular basis. These close ties may be maintained over time (Graham 1996, B1, B5).

Some solutions to loneliness and isolation may be unusual. Genevay (1993) describes a woman whose family relationships were painful. She dealt with the void in her life through involvement in the lives of soap opera characters. Other older people may try to establish family-like relationships with the professionals who work with them, with varying degrees of success. Professionals have to decide how to respond to this attempt to change the nature of their relationship. Computers and the Internet may offer nontraditional opportunities for older individuals, the disabled and homebound to develop new friends with whom they can communicate electronically in this technological age. Computers also offer a variety of educational and leisure activities, turning some users into information addicts.

Alone at the End: "I Never Thought it Would End Like This"

The quotation comes from my 87-year-old aunt when her doctor and those close to her concluded that she should no longer live alone. She had fallen one night when she was dizzy from the flu and had been unable to get up. She also was spending most of her time alone, although she had been very active before her husband died a few years earlier. The decision was difficult for all concerned. She had no children, so my sister and I took the initiative in finding a place we thought she would like. At first she was determined not to move, but seemed to realize that she should not be living alone any longer. Once she got used to the idea and visited several places, she settled comfortably in an attractive and well-run residence where she has a large room, filled with her own furniture, and a private bathroom. Other residents in the house are friendly and she soon was enjoying activities like playing bingo and exercise classes.

Many older women with no children or none living nearby will face similar decisions. Some will have adult children who are unwilling or unable to become caregivers and seek other arrangements. Sometimes the older person is the one who decides that she can no longer manage on her own. In other instances, relatives and friends will observe her difficulty in managing and suggest that a change is needed. Unfortunately, as indicated in chapter 4, the choices in appropriate places to live may be limited. Creative solutions are needed so that older women can live on their own and remain independent.

Ironically, after so many years of caring for children, parents and spouses, many women in their 70s and beyond find themselves without relatives or friends to care for them. This lack of relatives, friends or other support network, like a church group to provide care or companionship, poses special difficulties for poor or near-poor women in their last years. They cannot afford costly caregiving or household services. The solution for some is a nursing home, perhaps before they need that level of care.

The plight of elderly Chicago residents during the 1995 summer heat wave graphically demonstrates the difficulties. Hundreds of elderly persons died, largely because no one checked on them or because there was no place to send them for relief from the deadly temperatures.

Some retired adults are exploring alternatives to retirement communities and other formal institutional arrangements, preferring to live in a communal setting with other adults of the same age. Friedan describes some of these arrangements in *The Fountain of Age*. Maggie Kuhn of the Gray Panthers also advocated communal arrangements in which persons of various ages lived together. These informal arrangements may become more popular as active and healthy older Americans look for ways to share living space with others. Adults are making plans while they are independent for how they will live when they need assistance with daily living.

Some women want to make long-term care plans for when they may need it. A National Center for Women and Retirement Research publication, *Long Term Care for Women: How Will We Receive and Give Care*, provides planning information, including legal issues, insurance and advice for long-term caregivers. The suggestions are relevant to long-care needs of other family members as well. Advice for women planning for a spouse's long-term care without impoverishing themselves is helpful.

POLICIES TO IMPROVE WOMEN'S WELL-BEING AT MIDLIFE AND BEYOND

Improving Economic Security

As discussed in chapter 4, aging Americans are becoming a more diverse group. The 65-and-over population of the future will have more minorities and continued disproportionate numbers of women, especially among the "oldest old." Many will have limited or no assets as they approach retirement. Black and Hispanic females make up only 58 percent of the elderly population, but 74 percent of the elderly poor (Taeuber and Allen 1993, 23). If large numbers are not to spend their lives in poverty or near-poverty, then policies will have to change in three major areas: work and retirement; government entitlement programs such as Social Security and Medicare; and caregiving.

A frequent cause of poverty for an older women is the death of her spouse. She may be left with only a small income. She may have spent down their assets so that he qualified for Medicaid assistance in a nursing home or the cost of care may have depleted their assets. When family status and living arrangements are considered, the highest concentration of poverty is among older women living alone (Malveaux 1993, 174). ("Living alone" refers to those who are widowed, separated, divorced or never married.)

Work and Retirement

Women tend to be ignored or treated as adjuncts to their spouses when it comes to retirement policies and benefits. As noted earlier, they tend to earn less and are less likely to be covered by pensions (Hayward and Liu 1992, 22-23; OWL 1995).

Therefore, the basis of retirement policy, the "three-legged stool" of Social Security, employer pensions, and savings and investment, does not work well for women. "Unfortunately, caregiving, gender bias and lower women's wages translate into lower benefits later in life" (Glasse in OWL 1995, 6). Too many older women are poor because their primary or only income source is Social Security.

The higher national minimum wage will help to improve the lives of many low-income workers, both male and female. Women, who make up two-thirds of minimum-wage workers, especially benefit. Single women clearly will be better off. Moreover, the economic well-being of two-income families in which one or both spouses earn only the minimum wage will improve.

Other recommendations to improve women's economic status as workers include pay equity. Eleanor Holmes Norton introduced a Fair Pay Act: "Pay equity policy is an essential component of raising women's wages; equal opportunity and affirmative action alone are not sufficient" (quoted in Hartmann 1995, 16). Additionally, laws against age and race discrimination need strong enforcement.

Major policy changes also are needed with regard to retirement policies. Ways to do this include: giving benefits for unpaid work, earlier vesting of retirement benefits; more opportunities for workers to have IRAs and other investments; and mandated retirement credits for part-time workers. Many of these would benefit male or female low-income workers.

Private Pension Reform

The Women's Pension Policy Consortium, made up of the National Senior Citizens Law Center, the Older Women's League and the Pension Rights Center, began a campaign called "Pensions Not Posies" to increase public awareness of the important role pensions play in reducing women's poverty and to increase their participation in private pension plans. Only one-third of all retirees, and 23 percent of women, in this country receive such pensions.

Pension reform recommendations to benefit women include:

- make pensions mandatory for all employees, whether part-time or full-time workers and regardless of business size;
- reduce years required for vesting and allow nonvested workers who return after a break in service to resume progress toward vesting;
- make pensions portable so that workers who change jobs can move their pension benefit to a new job--a move in this direction occurred in 1996;
- add cost-of-living provisions to private sector pensions to reduce poverty among the oldest age groups, predominantly women;
- amend the Employees Retirement Income Security Act (ERISA) to specify that pensions, both vested and nonvested, are considered marital assets and can be divided (OWL 1995; Kuriansky 1994).

Social Security System Changes

The Social Security system, like the income tax system, is based on the "traditional" family model of the male worker with a stay-at-home wife. The majority of families do not fit this model. A married couple with two earners suffers a marriage penalty, paying more taxes than one with a single earner. Similarly, married women who contributed to the Social Security system over their work lives often get no greater benefit than does one who was never in the labor force (Hartmann 1995,15). However, one recent policy change increases a divorced woman's economic security by giving her the right to part of a ex-spouse's pension if they were married ten years or more.

Other suggested Social Security changes to improve the economic status of women, especially those who take time from the labor force for family responsibilities, include:

- Recognize differences in family arrangements, instead of using the stereotype of husband in the labor force and wife at home caring for the children.
- Give credit for caregiving responsibilities so that women are not penalized for years of caring for children and other family members.
- Give credit for unpaid work. Such a step seems unlikely, given current initiatives to cut health care costs by having families and volunteer groups assume more responsibility. *More* women may do *more* unpaid work.

Other Government Programs

Another frequently recommended change to benefit women is raising the Supplemental Security Income (SSI) benefit level to the poverty threshold (Davis et al. 1990, 199). Modifications to Medicare and Medicaid, especially sliding scale charges for purchasing benefits, would help older Americans, especially women.

Easing Caregiving Strains

The economic hardship of caring for family members, both young and old, has been a theme in this book. Family caregivers, usually women, are not compensated for their work. Hooyman (1992, 197) argues that caregiving should be given economic value, but the very words "care" and "giving" militate against defining it as "work." Government programs also tend to be directed toward helping only those who need care but don't have relatives to provide it (Davis et al. 1990). Otherwise, family members are expected to assume the responsibility for care, regardless of what it costs them.

Programs and policies are needed so that caregivers and recipients do not suffer undue economic hardship. Suggested changes include more alternatives to institutionalization, with an emphasis on helping the aging and the ill to remain at home with medical, household and supportive assistance for the caregiver.

Davis et al. (1990) recommend adding a new Medicare benefit to allow the severely impaired elderly to receive home care and adult day care services for a specified number of hours weekly. Such a provision would help many to avoid institutionalization and assist those most in need--those living alone, the poor and near-poor, and those who are most disabled. The caregivers also would get some time off.

Caregivers suffer financially in many ways. If they quit their job to look after an elderly relative, they lose not only income, but also their pension and other benefits. Women who change their schedule to work part-time also tend to be penalized. A Families and Work Institute study (1995, 12) found that only 30 percent of women working less than full-time had benefits, compared to 78 percent with full-time jobs.

The Family and Medical Leave Act allows family members to take time from their jobs temporarily to care for ill or elderly relatives. But they have to be able to afford to take this step. Policies also are needed to protect caregivers' retirement benefits when they take a leave. Scandinavian policies could provide a model, but the current political climate makes a move in that direction unlikely at this time (Hooyman 1992, 199).

The burdens on women as caregivers are not likely to be lightened until policies are no longer based on traditional views of the family, women's roles and government responsibility in this area (Seccombe 1992, 179). A concerted effort to increase men's participation in caregiving could focus on broadening their involvement from financial and home maintenance areas to other aspects of care (Marks 1993, 16). Such an approach would lighten the load on women, especially those who combine caregiving with labor force participation and other responsibilities (Hooyman; Seccombe; Marks). However, increased caregiving by males is unlikely until the pay gap between women and men narrows more. Women do the major part of the caregiving now because they lose less income than men do when they quit or decrease their hours of work. They are likely to continue to do so at least for the near future.

CHAPTER 6

Looking to the Future

POLICY ISSUES

The themes running through the previous chapters give rise to important policy issues for mid-life and older Americans in the future. As the twenty-first century approaches, these issues center around how individuals, families and society as a whole will deal with demographic and structural changes such as an aging American population and its growing diversity. A continuing and worrisome trend is the growing gap between the "haves" and the "have-nots." This gulf has been widening during the 1990s. The "haves" tend to be well-educated, have secure jobs with good benefits, and often belong to two-income households. The "have-nots" are disproportionately single individuals, especially female heads of households; the elderly or minorities; single males with limited education and job skills; and part-time, contingent or laid-off workers unable to find new jobs.

Structural changes in employment also will have a large impact on Americans at midlife in the future. An aging work force, job insecurity and a clouded outlook for young workers, especially the unskilled, will affect the well-being of future generations. A range of work-related policy issues under consideration at the national and state levels could improve prospects for all workers, young and old. The rise in the minimum wage, combined with the increased portability of pensions and portable health insurance, are changes that will benefit many Americans.

Because of their size, the baby-boom generation will have more influence than most other generations on the future. They may choose to be "silent" or politically active, but policy decisions affecting their own and their children's future will have to be made. Their views may reflect their experiences as "sandwich-generation" members, simultaneously rearing children and supporting aging parents (Bouvier and De Vita 1991, 31). The choices will not be easy. How will they balance their personal goals of achieving economic security against the needs of younger workers, including their own children, entering the labor force? Some self-interest may be involved in improving opportunities for young people since those who have trouble earning a living wage will have limited resources to help their parents in the future.

The costs of supporting older and younger Americans will be part of this public-policy debate. Parents pay a large part of the cost of child rearing, but the elderly get support from the federal government, supplemented by their own and their families' resources. A shifting of resources from services for the young to support increasing numbers of older persons raises questions about "public versus private responsibilities, as well as the appropriate level of government to address these needs" (Bouvier and De Vita 1991, 30).

As society confronts these issues, generational conflicts and tradeoffs may arise over setting priorities and allocating scarce resources. One way to resolve these tensions is by recognizing the interdependence of generations (Bouvier and De Vita 1991, 31). The challenge will be to devise policies that fairly allocate resources among age groups and balance the needs of older Americans with those of others, especially the young and the poor of all ages. Generational conflict has not erupted yet, but tensions may increase in the future as the cost of benefits for the elderly continues to rise and the need for choices becomes more evident (Toner 1995).

Studies show that Generation Xers do not expect to benefit from Social Security when they reach their 60s. A study of 18-to-34-year-olds found that 46 percent believe in UFOs, but only 28 percent expect Social Security to be around in their later years (Toner 1995). They expect the greatest strain on the system to occur when baby boomers retire (Romero 1994). At the same time, however, young and mid-life adults do not want to see benefits drastically cut for their older relatives. Moreover, many Generation Xers are showing concern for older relatives by caring for a grandparent. This represents a heavy burden for young adults who are just completing their education, getting established in the work force, or starting a family of their own.

This book has looked at how individuals and families deal with work and retirement, adult children who return to the nest, and aging parents. Although families often cope with difficult situations through trial-and-error informal arrangements, many issues require solutions at the societal level. However, if the past is a guide, major action is unlikely before issues become crises, since public policy almost always lags behind social needs (see Genovese 1984a).

New policies will be needed to deal with an aging workforce, the consequences of longer life expectancy for work and retirement; elder care; and inequalities that lead to a comfortable retirement for some and poverty for others. Moreover, strains between work and family responsibilities will continue to preoccupy workers, not only with regard to child care, but increasingly also elder care. As Americans live longer and perhaps work longer, they may find it more difficult to juggle these demands. The sheer numbers of aging Americans and the prevalence of two-worker and single-parent families will call for national solutions to replace the often ad hoc arrangements made by workers today. Some employers already are putting programs in place to ease workers' elder care responsibilities.

Emerging Trends in Work and Retirement

By the year 2030, projections indicate that more Americans will be over 65 than under 18 years of age. Baby boomers will comprise more than 50 percent of all workers. With fewer younger workers, employers may be more receptive to retaining or recruiting older employees. At present, only 12 percent of Americans aged 65 or older are in the labor force, either full- or part-time. Such a trend might decrease career opportunities for younger baby boomers and the baby-bust generation that followed (Bouvier and De Vita 27). Other factors working against older employees are the higher salaries they can command and the belief that they cannot adapt to technological change.

The End of Early Retirement?

It is likely to become harder for many Americans to retire early. Private pension plans fostered the trend toward early retirement in the past few decades (see chapter 2), yet these plans were confined largely to men, employees of larger companies, and those with higher education and earnings (Treas 1995, 28). Pensions also cover large numbers of public-sector workers who also had early retirement opportunities as governments sought to cut costs. Today, however, fewer mid-life or younger employees can rely on a fixed pension at retirement.

On average, Social Security provides the largest part (about 38 percent) of an older person's income, which often also is supplemented by personal assets and private pensions. But the solvency of the Social Security system for future retirees is debated today and surveys show that Generation Xers who followed baby boomers do not expect the system to be there for them (see Nelson and Cowan 1994).

The changing ratio of retirees to workers is a major concern, since the ratio of working-age to over-65 Americans is projected to drop from five-to-one in 1990 to three-to-one by the year 2030. Revisions made in 1983 to help control public costs of retirement will keep older workers on the job longer. Between the years 2000 and 2022, the retirement age for full Social Security benefits will rise from 65 to 67 years (Treas 1995, 24-25). More drastic measures may be needed to preserve the system, although opposition to controversial proposals will be widespread (see Peterson 1996). One recommendation is a means test for Social Security so that well-to-do Americans would be denied benefits. Other proposals are to allow the system to broaden its investment alternatives to include stocks or to allow workers to put part of their contributions in stocks and other investments. These approaches would change the nature of the system and might jeopardize payments to those older Americans whose only income comes from Social Security.

These uncertainties may make it harder for many baby boomers to retire early unless they have sufficient private resources. Their saving rates have been low and their debt high. Some experts predict a reversal in low savings rates as this generation begins to confront approaching retirement. However, circumstances beyond their control, including major economic disruptions, could interfere with planned savings.

Some individuals may choose to continue to work as long as they can. For example, "will their [divorced males] often lifelong isolation from former wives and children...prevent meaningful social relations during their retirement years and, perhaps, lead this group to delay retirement to maintain the social commerce that work provides?" (Szinovacz et al. 1992b, 260). Moreover, some younger baby boomers with limited educational and skill backgrounds and low incomes may not be able to think about retirement but will have to work as long as their health permits.

ELDER CARE: "WHO WILL LOOK AFTER US WHEN WE NEED IT?"

The meaning of old age is changing as more people stay healthy and active in their later years. In redefining "old," gerontologists often divide this period into two or even three categories, differentiating between the "young-old," who are active and in good health, and the "old-old," those over age 85 (Skolnick 1991, 163). Differing viewpoints exist about the health of the oldest group. Some experts expect this group to suffer from chronic and debilitating diseases, especially Alzheimer's disease, while others insist that they tend to be in good health, having avoided many chronic diseases that cause death at earlier ages. They suggest that the oldest-old are more likely to die after a short illness.

Nonetheless, by 80 years of age, many individuals will experience health problems, have difficulty with daily tasks, and become more dependent on others. Mid-life adults may find their years of caregiving extended as parents live longer (Hayward and Liu 1992, 49-50).

This experience may make baby boomers fear that they may require more years of care than their parents will and worry about how they will get it. In 1992, for example, almost 16 percent of those aged 40-44 had no children. Compared to their parents, a higher proportion is likely to be childless. Moreover, the number of older Americans who are alone continues to increase and many are low-income women, as the discussion in chapter 5 indicates. With a small number of potential caregivers, the elderly in the next century will rely more on costly formal services (Treas 1995, 29).

However, young family members may step in to assist their older relatives. A recent study found that Generation Xers already were assuming caregiving responsibilities. A survey by the National Council on the Aging and John Hancock Mutual Life Insurance found that a surprisingly high proportion of adults under the age of 32 years, 24 percent, either were giving or had given long-term care to a family member or friend. The comparable figure for the general population is 24 percent (Shellenbarger 1996).

This group of mid-life Americans also is unique because high rates of divorce and remarriage create ambiguity about the roles their children will adopt vis-à-vis divorced parents. Will the adult children of divorced parents assume responsibility for *both* parents, or only the one who raised them? In acrimonious divorces, one partner may be shunned by the children who sided with the other parent. Will they provide day-to-day care or contribute to the costs of paid care for either parent? We also can ask whether adult children are likely to become caregivers to step-parents; their decision will depend in part on how close their relationship was. The answers to these questions will affect care for many older Americans (Bouvier and De Vita 1991, 31).

Consequently, caring for older Americans will be a major issue for families and for society as a whole in the next century. Despite policy-makers' discussions about ways to provide long-term care, there is no assurance that universal health and long-term care programs will be enacted in the near future. Alternatives being considered include some form of government insurance for long-term institutional care or funding of long-term in-home services for the elderly. Spiraling health care costs for the elderly ultimately may result in a national health care system for all Americans, young and old. The need for health care access spans the generations, but the young are often most disadvantaged. Recent cuts in health care have been directed toward the poor and children, rather than the elderly. Making preventive health care available to all Americans might become accepted as a way to cut down on costly medical care for untreated and avoidable medical conditions.

Quality of Life Issues

It seems inevitable that the quality of life for those living into their late 80s and beyond will become a subject of debate. Those who need a high level of care will be in nursing homes, especially if no close relatives are able to provide care. Anyone visiting a nursing home or the geriatric floor of a hospital cannot help but ask about the benefits of living to a "ripe old age." Older persons can be kept alive by complicated combinations of medication and treatments, but their lives provide few satisfactions and little enjoyment. Euthanasia and doctor-assisted suicide will be debated increasingly as Americans' life spans are extended with no accompanying improvement in their quality of life.

For those in their 70s or older and in good health, more alternative living arrangements clearly are needed. More experiments will be tried that will allow individuals to stay in their own homes with services provided. Community services like adult day care can eliminate some of the isolation of older persons, by offering activities, companionship and a way to monitor their health, nutrition and daily functioning. Informal arrangements of congenial older persons who decide to live together may become more common. Some areas have registries designed to link up compatible elderly persons with each other or with households. As these arrangements become more prevalent, the need for oversight will grow, since the potential for mistreatment or for inadequate facilities exists.

Elder abuse is a growing concern. It can be found in informal settings, in which caregivers are either relatives or paid aides, or in institutional settings (see AARP 1992a and b; Steinmetz 1988). It is often hidden and difficult to verify because the elderly individual comes into contact with few people other than the caregiver. It also may not be recognized because frail elderly persons, especially those with osteoporosis, have frequent falls and fractured bones. More oversight of institutions large and small is needed. The medical profession also should become increasingly alert to evidence of mistreatment of elderly patients and quicker to report instances of suspected abuse.

CHANGE AND THE RESILIENCE OF FAMILIES

In the face of complex situations, members have shown resiliency in dealing with issues ranging from planning for retirement or surviving layoffs, to coping with "boomerang" adult children who return home, or assuming responsibility for aging parents who need care in their later years. Mid-life individuals will continue to meet the needs of younger and older family members, even when it means giving up or postponing their own plans and priorities. Moreover, despite the frequent claims that the family is dead, made by politicians fixated on the idealized 1950s television version of the family, American families continue to be an anchor for their members even as their composition and relationships become more diverse.

Individuals are redefining what constitutes a family in their own lives but, at the societal level, strong disagreements exist about how or even whether public policy should reflect such changes (see Skolnick 1991; Goldscheider and Waite 1991; and Popenoe 1988). For example, government and employer benefits for cohabiting unmarried individuals, whether homosexual or heterosexual, represent one area in which policy is changing, despite opposition from conservative groups; many large employers now extend benefits to employees in such relationships.

In recognition of the high divorce rate in our society, ex-spouses now have legal claims to their former partner's pension under certain conditions. This right is especially important to mid-life women who may be divorced after twenty-five or more years of marriage. High divorce and remarriage rates, especially among Americans in their young adult and middle years, will have an economic and social impact in later life and may affect the life chances of their children.

Americans with former and current families at midlife have varying degrees of closeness and interaction with members. If both spouses were married previously and have children, relationships are even more complicated. After family members divorce and remarry, individuals and families are faced with working out appropriate behavior or "etiquette" with former relatives.

There is no clear precedent for deciding how to relate to ex-relatives after divorce. The individuals concerned have to decide whether or not to maintain ties. Some may cut off all contact with families of their former spouses, much to the dismay and anguish of grandparents who often seek legal means to obtain visitation rights in the courts; while others continue to see former relatives and to consider them still "family."

Families will continue to struggle with the ever-changing responsibilities and demands on members, rearranging schedules and adding on duties. Support from other institutions in society, especially government and work, could make it easier for them to manage multiple responsibilities. The issues and needs are well-defined, but differing viewpoints about the definition and meaning of "family" make solutions in the form of public policies and programs difficult to attain. Women may make a difference as they occupy more positions of power and play a larger role in setting policy in both government and work organizations. Since they are the "kinkeepers," they have a special interest in working for change to improve the well-being of mid-life Americans and families in general.

Appendix A: Organizations, Support Groups, and Other Resources

Alliance for Aging Research
2021 K St. NW
Suite 305
Washington, DC 20006
(202) 293-2856
> Promotes research on aging and offers informational booklets.

American Association of Homes and Services for the Aging
Communications Department
901 E. Street NW, Suite 500
Washington, DC 20004
(202) 783-2242; (800) 675-9253
> Free brochures on choosing a nursing home or assisted-living facility. Also provides a directory of retirement communities with continuing care and advice on insurance for long-term care.

American Association of Individual Investors
625 North Michigan Avenue
Chicago, Illinois 60611
(312) 280-0170
> An independent, not-for-profit corporation that helps individuals manage their assets more effectively through educational programs, information and research. Subscription to *The Individual Investor*, published five times a year, is $13. Also publishes books and reports on such topics as no-load mutual funds and computerized investing.

American Association of Retired Persons (AARP)
601 East Street, NW
Washington, DC 20049
(800) 424-3410

Publications on retirement planning, health, housing, and financial planning, including *Modern Maturity* and *Working Age*. Also does advocacy on issues relating to aging, older workers and retirement. Members get discounts on various products.

American Association of Retired Persons (AARP)
Grandparent Information Center
601 East Street, NW
Washington, DC 20049
Telephone: (202) 434-2296, Monday to Friday, 9 a.m. to 5 p.m.
FAX: (202) 434-6474

Connects grandparents with local support groups and resources. Works with national and local agencies involved in child care, aging issues, and legal and family services. (Received more than 4,700 calls for help in 1993.)

American Bar Association--Commission on Legal Problems of the Elderly
1604 North Country Club Road
Tucson, AZ 85716
(602) 881-4005

Offers a booklet on selecting an elder law attorney. Send a legal-sized self-addressed envelope.

American Self-Help Clearinghouse
25 Pocono Road
Denville, NJ 07834
Telephone: (201) 625-7101
TDD Line: (201) 625-9053
FAX: (201) 625-8848

Provides a listing of national and local self-help support groups for illness, disability, bereavement or other stresses.

Children of Aging Parents (CAPS)
1609 Woodbourne Road
Department P, Suite 302-A
Levittown, PA 19057
Telephone: (215) 945-6900; (800) 227-7294
FAX: (215) 945-8720

A national clearinghouse for caregivers of the elderly and for professionals in the field of aging. Offers a variety of materials, including manuals, newsletters and fact sheets. Prepares a national directory of support groups for caregivers of the elderly and offers telephone counseling.

Choice in Dying
200 Varick Street
New York, NY 10014
(800) 989-9455
    A nonprofit organization offering assistance to the dying and their relatives. Makes living will and health proxy forms available.

Continuing Care Accreditation Commission
901 E Street NW, Suite 500
Washington, DC 20004
Telephone: (202) 783-7286
FAX: (202) 783-2255
    This commission accredits both for-profit and not-for-profit retirement communities offering continuing care. Has lists of accredited housing by area.

Displaced Homemakers Network
1411 K Street, NW, Suite 930
Washington, DC 20005
(202) 628-6767
    Programs provide training, counseling and referrals to other community resources for women entering or returning to the labor force after many years, especially after divorce or widowhood.

Eldercare America
1141 Loxford Terrace
Silver Spring, MD 20901
(301) 593-1621
    Information on elder care workshops and videotapes for sale.

Eldercare Locator
National Association of Area Agencies on Aging
(800) 677-1116
    A federally funded network of 675 area agencies on aging. Provides free information and referrals on aging services throughout the United States. A local resource and referral organization has information on such services as assisted-living facilities and home health care aides or other support for elderly persons living at home. Services are not screened by the agency.

The Family Caregiver Alliance
(formerly The Family Survival Project)
425 Bush Street, Suite 500
San Francisco, CA 94108
(415) 434-3388 (out-of-state); (800) 445-8106 (California)
    Information for families and caregivers of brain-impaired adults.

Family Enterprises
11700 West Lake Park Drive
Milwaukee, WI 53224
Telephone: (414) 359-1055
FAX: (414) 359-1074
   Publishes a newsletter, *Eldercare Connection*, for employees who provide care for elderly relatives. Services include a consultation and referral program and caregiver support group.

Family Service America
11700 West Lake Park Drive
Milwaukee, WI 53224
Telephone: (414) 359-1040; (800) 221-2681
FAX: (414) 359-1074
   A national organization that assists individuals and families.

Federation of Parents and Friends of Lesbians and Gays, Inc.
P.O. Box 24565
Los Angeles, CA 90024

Foundation for Hospice and Home Care
519 C Street NE
Washington, DC 20002
(202) 547-6586
   Send a stamped, self-addressed business envelope for free publications.

GAP (Grandparents as Parents)
P. O. Box 964
Lakewood, CA 90714
(310) 924-3996
   A nonprofit clearinghouse linking grandparents to support groups across the country.

Grandparents Raising Grandchildren
Barbara Kirkland
P.O. Box 104
Colleyville, TX 76034
(817) 577-0435

Grandparents United for Children's Rights
137 Larkin Street
Madison, WI 53705
(608) 238-8751
   Focuses on the needs of custodial grandparents and those who want more access to their grandchildren. Provides information on local chapters and information on state laws relating to custody and visitation.

Gray Panthers
2025 Pennsylvania Avenue NW, Suite 821
Washington, DC 20006
(202) 466-3132

Works on problems of the elderly, especially health care, affordable housing and equity issues. Publishes a newsletter and reports on legislation. Local chapters are found across the country.

Health Insurance Association of America
1025 Connecticut Avenue NW, Suite 1200
Washington, DC 20036
National Insurance Consumer Helpline: (800) 942-4242

Offers information and publications on health insurance, including *A Consumer's Guide to Medicare Insurance* and *A Consumer's Guide to Long-Term Care Insurance.*

Institute for Women's Policy Research (IWPR)
1400 20th Street NW, Suite 104
Washington, DC 20036
Telephone: (202) 785-5100
FAX: (202) 833-4362

Publishes research, policy statements and reports in areas such as women's employment and careers, income and poverty, health and related topics.

Institute of Certified Financial Planners
7600 East Eastman Avenue, Suite 301
Denver, CO 80231
(800) 282-7526, Monday to Friday, 8 a.m. to 5 p.m., Mountain Time

Provides names and qualifications of several certified financial planners in your area and a brochure on how to select a planner.

International Association for Financial Planning
2 Concourse Parkway, Suite 800
Atlanta, GA 30328
(404) 395-1605

Legal Services Corporation
750 First Street NE
Washington, DC 20002
(202) 336-8800

National Accessible Apartment Clearinghouse
(800) 421-1221

Keeps a record of apartments accessible to the disabled in metropolitan areas across the country. There is no charge for referrals or for listing an apartment.

National Alliance for Caregiving
7201 Wisconsin Avenue, Suite 620
Bethesda, MD 20814
Telephone: (301) 718-8444
FAX: (301) 718-0034
A new national resource center for caregivers to the elderly resulting from a partnership of four organizations--the American Society on Aging, the National Council on the Aging, the National Association of Area Agencies on Aging, and the Department of Veterans Affairs; funded by Glaxo-Welcome. Offers fact sheets and resources lists on caregiving.

National Association for Home Care
529 C Street NE, Stanton Park
Washington, DC 20002
Telephone: (202) 547-7424
FAX: (202) 547-3540

A national organization for the home health care field whose interests include advocacy, policy and education. Provides a brochure, "How to Choose a Home Care Agency."

National Association of Area Agencies on Aging
1112 16th Street NW, Suite 100
Washington, DC 20036
(202) 296-8130
Has programs in every state. Many are subsidized and free; others have a sliding scale or are covered by Medicaid (Title XIX).

National Association of Investors Corp.
P.O. Box 220
Royal Oak, MI 48068
(810) 583-6242
Provides information on investment clubs and also offers a chat room on the Web (see below).

National Association of Personal Financial Advisors
1130 West Lake Cook Road, Suite 150
Buffalo Grove, IL 60089
Telephone: (708) 537-7722; (800) 366-2732
FAX: (708) 537-7740
Provides a list of fee-only financial planners in your area and a form to use when interviewing planners.

National Association of Professional Geriatric Care Managers
1604 North Country Club Road
Tucson, AZ 85716
Telephone: (520) 881-8008
FAX: (520) 325-7925
     Provides referrals and information on hiring a manager in your community.

National Association of State Units on Aging
(202) 898-2578
     Provides referrals to the caller's state agency.

National Center and Caucus on Black Aging
1424 K Street NW, Suite 500
Washington, DC 20005
(202) 637-8400
     Has a program to place those 55 years or older in jobs and provides training and development for minorities in nursing home administration.

National Center for Women and Retirement Research
Long Island University
Southampton, NY 11968
(800) 426-7386
     A university-based center that focuses on life planning for women and studies the financial needs of mid-life women. Publishes reports and life planning handbooks on finances and social, emotional, health and care issues for mid-life women. Also has seminars and videotapes.

National Center on Elder Abuse
810 First Street NE
Washington, DC 20002
Telephone: (202) 682-2470
FAX: (202) 289-6555

National Citizens Coalition for Nursing Home Reform
1424 16th Street NW, Suite 202
Washington, DC 20036
Telephone: (202) 332-2275
FAX: (202) 332-2949
     An advocacy group that works for nursing home reforms and provides consumer information.

National Coalition Against Domestic Violence
2401 Virginia Avenue NW, Suite 306
Washington, DC 20037
(202) 638-6388

National Coalition of Grandparents
137 Larkin Street
Madison, WI 53705
(608) 238-8751
> Works for changes in legislation at the national and state levels.

National Committee for the Prevention of Elder Abuse
119 Belmont Street
Worcester, MA 01605
Telephone: (508) 793-6166
FAX: (508) 793-6906
> Helps in forming affiliate groups and developing prevention programs. Provides information and referrals, and publishes the *Journal of Elder Abuse and Neglect*.

National Consumer League
1701 K Street NW, Suite 1200
Washington, DC 20006
Telephone: (202) 835-3323
FAX: (202) 835-0747
> Provides information on food and drug safety, medical care costs, consumer and telecommunications fraud.

National Council on the Aging
409 Third Street SW, Suite 200
Washington, DC 20024
(202) 479-1200
> Provides free pamphlets on caregiving and family home care and referrals to local service agencies. The organization includes the National Institute of Senior Centers and the National Institute of Adult Day Care, and the National Institute on Financial Issues, and Services for Elders.

National Eldercare Institute
University of South Florida
Suncoast Gerontology Center
12901 Bruce B. Downs Boulevard, MDC Box 50
Tampa, FL 33613
(813) 974-4355; (800) 633-4563 (in Florida only)
> Referrals to programs in Florida and national information on long-term care.

National Family Caregivers Association
9223 Longbranch Parkway
Silver Spring, MD 20901
(301) 949-3638

National Foundation for Consumer Credit
8701 Georgia Avenue, Suite 601
Silver Spring, MD 20910
(301) 589-5600
> Will refer a caller to a counseling service in their area.

National Hispanic Council on Aging
2713 Ontario Road NW, Suite 200
Washington, DC 20009
(202) 265-1288
> Provides resources for and about older Hispanics.

National Hospice Organization
1901 North Moore Street, Suite 901
Arlington, VA 22209
Telephone: (703) 243-5900
Referral Helpline: (800) 638-8898, Monday to Friday, 8:30 a.m. to 5:30 p.m.,
Eastern time

National Indian Council on Aging
P.O. Box 2088
Albuquerque, NM 87110
(505) 242-9505
> The Council's membership supports older Indians and offers resource
information for older Native Americans.

National Institute on Aging
(800) 222-2225
> Offers free materials on such topics as medication, safety and nutrition.
For publications, write: Public Information Office, Federal Building, 6th Floor,
Bethesda, MD 20892.

National Pacific/Asian Resource Center on Aging
1511 Third Avenue, Suite 914
Seattle, WA 98101
(206) 448-0313
> Provides information about older Pacific/Asian individuals.

National Self-Help Clearinghouse
33 West 42nd Street
New York, NY 10036
(212) 354-8525
> Gives information and referrals to support groups.

National Senior Citizens Law Center (NSCLC)
1815 H Street NW, Suite 700
Washington, DC 20006
(202) 887-5280
        Offers technical assistance to lawyers who represent older workers, retirees and beneficiaries on pension matters. As a Legal Services Corporation back-up center, NSCLC does not aid individuals but will provide referrals.

National Support Center for Families of the Aging
(215) 544-5933

Older Women's League (OWL)
666 11th Street NW
Washington, DC 20001
(202) 783-6686; (800) 825-3695
        Advocacy group for mid-life and older women, especially concerning pensions and job opportunities. Has about 120 chapters across the country.

Pension Rights Center
918 16th Street NW, Suite 704
Washington, DC 20006
(202) 296-3776
        Nonprofit organization that works to safeguard pension rights of workers, retirees and their families. Projects include the Women's Pension Project, the National Pension Assistance Project and the Technical Assistance Project. Provides information about pension issues.

ROCKING (Raising Our Children's Kids: An Intergenerational Network of Grandparenting)
Mary Fron
P.O. Box 96
Niles, MI 49120
(616) 683-9038

The Rosalynn Carter Institute for Human Development
Georgia Southwestern College
800 Wheatley Street
Americus, GA 31709
(912) 928-1234

SeniorNet
399 Arguello Boulevard
San Francisco, CA 94118
(415) 750-5030
        Provides computer education to older adults. Membership costs $25 annually and includes a newsletter and discounts on various items. Also has an on-line service.

Service Corps of Retired Executives (SCORE)
(National office) 409 Third Street SW, Suite 5900
Washington, DC 20024
(202) 205-6762
Chapters of retired business people across the country volunteer to help small businesses with training and advice. Information on the program also is available from the Small Business Administration.

Social Security Administration (SSA)
Office of Public Inquiries
6401 Security Boulevard
Baltimore, MD 21235
(410) 965-1234; (800) 772-1213

U.S. Department of Labor
Pension and Welfare Benefit Administration
200 Constitution Avenue NW
Washington, DC 20210
For information about your rights under federal private pension laws, call (202) 219-8776. For copies of summary plan descriptions and pension financial reports, call (202) 219-8771. For copies of *How to File a Claim for Benefits, How to Obtain Employee Benefit Documents from the Labor Department, What You Should Know About the Pension Law,* and other booklets on employee benefits, write to the Labor Department, Room N-55211, at the above address.

U.S. Equal Employment Opportunity Commission (EEOC)
1801 L Street NW
Washington, DC 20507
(202) 663-4900
Call 800-USA-EEOC to register a complaint or report it to your local office.

Visiting Nurse Association
3801 East Florida Avenue, Suite 900
Denver, CO 80210
Telephone: (303) 753-0218; (800) 426-2547
FAX: (303) 753-0258
A national organization that provides referrals to the local organizations providing nonprofit health care services in cities and rural areas. Services include various types of therapy and other services.

Appendix B: Computer Software and On-line Services

FINANCIAL SOFTWARE

Financial planning and money management software is available at computer stores. Two of the most widely used programs are:

- **Managing Your Money**
  (800) 624-9060

- **Quicken Personal Finance**
  (800) 537-9993

FINANCIAL INFORMATION ON THE INTERNET

On-line and Internet financial information sources are growing with new Web sites for financial planning, investing and related topics appearing daily. On-line trading possibilities also are proliferating. Some places to start for information on financial topics include the following:

- **American Association of Individual Investors** (Keyword: AAII) has a forum on America Online with articles from their publications, information about investment resources in the reference library, demos and spreadsheets for downloading. Users also can post messages on investment topics.

- **America Online** offers a variety of other resources, including Morningstar's profiles of mutual funds and Wall Street Words for definitions of investment terms.

- **Compuserve** offers several free financial services: *Money Magazine's* Fund-Watch Online with data on almost 2,000 mutual funds, the "Investor's Forum," and a chat room by the National Association of Investors Corporation, an organization of investment clubs.

- **NETworth** (http://networth.galt.com), a personal finance site on the Web, provides information on mutual funds, including data from Morningstar and current net asset values.

ELECTRONIC JOB HUNTING

The growing number of on-line services includes:

- **America's Employers**-- http://www.americasemployers.com
- **America's Job Bank**-- http://www.ajb.dni.us
- **CareerMosaic**-- http://www.careermosaic.com
- **CareerPath**-- http://www.careerpath.com
- **CareerSite**--http://www.careersite.com
- **Career City**-- http://www.careercity.com
- **Career Magazine Database**-- http://www.careermag.com
- **E-Span**-- http://www.espan.com
- **Help Wanted USA**-- http://www.iccweb.com
- **The MonsterBoard**-- http://www.monster.com
- **NationJob Network**-- http://www.nationjob.com
- **Online Career Center**-- http://www.occ.com

RETIREMENT AND CAREGIVING TOPICS

Those seeking information on these topics might start with the following:

- **America Online**
(800) 827-6364
Better Health and Medical Forum topics include "Seniors' Health and Caregiving." Articles can be downloaded or read on-line.

- **Compuserve**
(800) 848-8199
Retirement Living Forum includes such topics as "Caregiving" and "Town Square," a social area. The information can be downloaded from the electronic bulletin board. The chance to chat on-line with others can serve as a support group for users, especially for those who would find it difficult to attend meetings outside the house.

- **AARP information**
On CompuServe, Go-AARP provides information and interactive forums on issues of interest to those over 50 years of age. On America Online, Keyword: AARP, Thursday chats with AARP staff member and guests are available. On Prodigy, Jump: AARP, has AARP staff members on Wednesday night in the Member Coffee Shop from 9 to 10 p.m. All three services carry articles from the AARP *Bulletin*.

Information on housing and care options for older persons is available from a Web site of the California Association of Homes and Services for the Aging at www.seniorsites.com.

Bibliography

GENERAL BOOKS, ARTICLES AND REPORTS

Abel, E. 1986. "Adult Daughters and Care for the Elderly." *Feminist Studies* 12: 279-497.

Abel, Emily. 1994. *Who Cares for the Elderly? Public Policy and the Experiences of Adult Daughters.* Philadelphia, PA: Temple University Press.

Ahlburg, Dennis A. and Carol J. De Vita. 1992. "New Realities of the American Family." *Population Bulletin* 47, 2 (August).

Aldous, Joan. 1995. "New Views on Grandparents in Intergenerational Context." *Journal of Family Issues* 16, 1 (January): 104-122.

Aldous, J. and D. M. Klein. 1991. "Sentiment and Services: Models of Intergenerational Relationships in Mid-life." *Journal of Marriage and the Family* 53 (August): 595-608.

Allen, Jessie. 1993a. "The Front Lines." Pp. 1-10 in *Women on the Front Lines: Meeting the Challenge of an Aging America.* Washington, DC: Urban Institute Press.

Allen, Jessie. 1993b. "Caring Work and Gender Equity in an Aging Society." Pp. 221-239 in *Women on the Front Lines: Meeting the Challenge of an Aging America.* Washington, DC: Urban Institute Press.

Allen, Jessie and Alan Pifer (eds.). 1993. *Women on the Front Lines: Meeting the Challenge of an Aging America.* Washington, DC: Urban Institute Press.

American Association of Retired Persons (AARP). 1991a. "The Contingent Workforce: Implications for Midlife and Older Women." Fact Sheet. Women's Initiative, AARP.

American Association of Retired Persons. 1992a. *Abused Elders or Older Battered Women?* Report on the AARP Forum, Washington, DC, October 29-30, 1992.

American Association of Retired Persons. 1992b. *Domestic Mistreatment of the Elderly: Towards Prevention.* Prepared for AARP by Richard L. Douglass.

American Association of Retired Persons. 1994a. "Employed Caregivers Experience Both Stress and Rewards." *Working Age* 10, 4 (November/December): 5-7.

American Association of Retired Persons. 1995. "Many Employers Help Working Caregivers by Offering Dependent Care Assistance Plans." *Working Age* 11, 4 (November/December): 4-5.

American Association of Retired Persons and Travelers Companies Foundation. 1988. *National Survey of Caregivers: Summary of Findings.* Washington, DC: AARP.

Anderson, K. L. and W. R. Allen. 1984. "Correlates of Extended Household Structure." *Phylon* 45 (2): 144-157.

Angel, R. and M. Tienda. 1982. "Determinants of Extended Family Structure: Cultural Pattern or Economic Need?" *American Journal of Sociology* 87: 1360-1383.

Aquilino, W. S. and K. R. Supple. 1991. "Parent-Child Relations and Parents' Satisfaction When Adult Children Live at Home." *Journal of Marriage and the Family* 53 (February): 13-28.

Barnett, R. C., N. Kibria, G. K. Baruch, and J. H. Pleck. 1991. "Adult Daughter-Parent Relations and Daughter's Well-Being." *Journal of Marriage and the Family* 53 (February): 29-42.

Barresi, Charles M. and Geeta Menon. 1990. "Diversity in Black Family Caregiving." Pp. 221-235 in *Black Aged: Understanding Diversity and Service Needs*, Zev Harel, Edward A. McKinney, and Michael Williams, eds. Newbury Park, CA: Sage Publications.

Bengtsen, V. L. and J. F. Robertson (eds.). 1985. *Grandparenthood: Research and Policy Perspectives.* Beverly Hills, CA: Sage Publications.

Bennefield, Robert L. 1996. "Who Loses Coverage and for How Long?" U.S. Bureau of the Census. *Current Population Reports.* Household Economic Studies P70-54. May.

Bianchi, Suzanne M. 1987. "Living at Home: Young Adults' Living Arrangements in the 1980s." Paper presented at the Annual Meeting of the American Sociological Association in Chicago.

Blankenhorn, David, Steven Bayme, and Jean Bethke Elshtain (eds.). 1990. *Rebuilding the Nest: A New Commitment to the American Family.* Milwaukee, WI: Family Service America.

Booth, Alan and Paul R. Amato. 1994. "Parental Marital Quality, Parental Divorce and Relations with Parents." *Journal of Marriage and the Family* 56 (February): 21-34.

Bouvier, Leon F. and Carol J. De Vita. 1991. "The Baby Boom--Entering Midlife." *Population Bulletin* 46, 3 (November).

Boyd, Monica and Edward T. Pryor. 1988. "The Cluttered Nest: The Living Arrangements of Young Canadian Adults." Paper presented at the annual meetings of the Canadian Population Society and Canadian Sociological and Anthropological Association. Windsor, Ontario, Canada.

Brody, E. 1985. "Parent Care as a Normative Family Stress." *The Gerontologist* 25: 19-29.

Brody, Elaine M., Christine Hoffman, Morton H. Kleban, and Claire B. Schoonover. 1989. "Caregiving Daughters and their Local Siblings: Perceptions, Strains, and Interactions." *The Gerontologist* 29: 529-538.

Brody, Elaine. 1990. *Women in the Middle: Their Parent-Care Years*. New York: Springer Publishing Co.

Brody, E., S. Litvin, C. Hoffman, and M. Kleban. 1992. "Differential Effects of Daughters' Marital Status on Their Parent Care Experiences." *The Gerontologist* 32: 58-67.

Brubaker, Timothy H. 1985. *Later Life Families.* Newbury Park, CA: Sage Publications.

Brubaker, Timothy H. (ed.) 1990. *Family Relationships in Later Life,* 2nd Ed. Newbury Park, CA: Sage Publications.

Brubaker, Ellie and Timothy H. Brubaker. 1992. "The Context of Retired Women as Caregivers." Pp. 222-235 in *Families and Retirement,* Maximiliane Szinovacz, David J. Ekerdt and Barbara H. Vinick, eds. Newbury Park, CA: Sage Publications.

Bumpass, Larry and William S. Aquilino. 1995. *A Social Map of Midlife: Family and Work Over the Middle Life Course.* The MacArthur Foundation Research Network on Successful Midlife Development. March.

Burton, Linda M. 1992. "Black Grandparents Rearing Children of Drug-Addicted Parents: Stressors, Outcomes, and Social Service Needs." *The Gerontologist* 32: 744-751.

Burton, Linda M. (ed.). 1993. *Families and Aging.* Generations and Aging Series. Amityville, NY: Baywood Publishing.

Burton, Linda M. and Cynthia de Vries. 1993. "Challenges and Rewards: African-American Grandparents as Surrogate Parents." Pp. 101-108 in *Families and Aging,* Linda Burton, ed. Amityville, NY: Baywood Publishing.

Burton, L. M. and P. Dilworth-Anderson. 1991. "The Intergenerational Roles of Aged Black Americans." *Marriage and Family Review* 16: 311-331.

Carpenter, Liz. 1994a. "Liz's Excellent Adventure In Which a 70 Year Old Widow Takes on a Houseful of Teenagers." *Modern Maturity* (November-December): 38, 40, 41.

Chalfie, Deborah. 1994. *Going It Alone: A Closer Look at Grandparents Parenting Grandchildren.* Washington, DC: American Association of Retired Persons.

Chudacoff, Howard and Tamara Hareven. 1979. "From Empty Nest to Family Dissolution: Life Course Transitions into Old Age." *Journal of Family History* 4: 69-83.

Cicirelli, Victor. 1983. "A Comparison of Helping Behavior to Elderly Parents of Adult Children with Intact and Disrupted Marriages." *The Gerontologist* 23: 619-625.

Clignet, R. 1992. *Death, Deeds and Descendants: Inheritance in Modern America.* Hawthorne, NY: Aldine.

Climo, Jacob. 1992. *Distant Parents.* New Brunswick, NJ: Rutgers University Press.

Coberly, Sally and Gail G. Hunt. 1995. "The Metlife Study of Employer Costs for Working Caregivers." Prepared for Senior Services Division, Metropolitan Life Insurance Company. Washington, DC: Washington Business Group on Health.

Cochran, Moncrieff, et al. 1990. *Extending Families: The Social Networks of Parents and their Children.* New York: Cambridge University Press.

Cole, Al. 1995. "From a Distance." *Modern Maturity* (March-April): 92-93.

Conaway, James. 1996. "Reinventing the Good Life." *Fortune* (August 19): 110-118.

Congressional Budget Office, Congress of the United States. 1993. *Baby Boomers in Retirement: An Early Perspective.* September.

Corporate Benefits Institute. 1994. *Dependent Care Assistance Programs (DCAPs): Survey Results.* December. Brookfield, WI: International Foundation of Employee Benefit Plans.

Coward, R. T., C. Horne, and J. W. Dwyer. 1992. "Demographic Perspectives on Gender and Family Caregiving." Pp. 18-33 in *Gender, Families, and Elder Care,* J. W. Dwyer and R. T. Coward, eds. London: Sage Publications.

Crimmins, Eileen and Dominique Ingegneri. 1990. "Interaction and Living Arrangements of Older Parents and their Children." *Research on Aging* 12: 158-181.

Crittenden, Ann. 1994. "Temporary Solutions." *Working Woman* (February): 32-35, 71.

Cronin, Roberta and Juanda Kirk. 1991. *The Financial Impact of Multiple Family Responsibilities on Midlife and Older People: An Exploratory Study.* Washington, DC: AARP.

Crowley, Susan L. 1993. "Grandparents to the Rescue." *AARP Bulletin* (October): 1, 16.

Crowley, Susan L. and Leah K. Glasheen. 1996. *AARP Bulletin* (February): 1, 12, 13.

Cumming, Elaine and William Henry. 1961. *Growing Old: The Process of Disengagement.* New York: Basic Books.

DaVanzo, Julie and Frances Goldscheider. 1990. "Coming Home Again: Returns to the Nest in Young Adulthood." *Population Studies* 44, 2(July): 241-255.

Davis, Karen, Paula Grant, and Diane Rowland. 1990. "Alone and Poor: The Plight of Elderly Women." *Generations: Gender and Aging* (Summer): 43-47.

Day, Jennifer Cheeseman. 1996. "Projections of the Number of Households and Families in the United States: 1995-2010." U.S. Bureau of the Census, *Current Population Reports*, P25-1129. Washington, DC: U.S. Government Printing Office.

Dechter, Aimée and Pamela J. Smock. 1994. "The Fading Breadwinner Role and the Economic Implications for Young Couples." Institute for Research on Poverty Discussion Papers. University of Wisconsin-Madison. December.

Delany, Sarah L. and A. Elizabeth Delany, with Amy Hill Heath. 1994. *Having Our Say: The Delany Sisters' First Hundred Years.* New York: Dell.

Dilworth-Anderson, Peggye. 1993. "Extended Kin Networks in Black Families." Pp. 57-65 in *Families and Aging*, Linda Burton, ed. Amityville, NY: Baywood Publishing Company.

Dwyer, Jeffrey W. and Raymond T. Coward (eds.). 1992. *Gender, Families, and Elder Care.* Newbury Park, CA: Sage Publications.

Dwyer, Jeffrey W., Gary R. Lee, and Thomas B. Jankowski. 1994. "Reciprocity, Elder Satisfaction, and Caregiver Stress and Burden: The Exchange of Aid in the Family Caregiving Relationship." *Journal of Marriage and the Family* 56, 1 (February): 35-43.

Eggebeen, D. J. and D. P. Hogan. 1990. "Giving Between the Generations in American Families." *Human Nature* 1: 211-32.

Eller, T. J. 1994. "Household Wealth and Asset Ownership: 1991." U.S. Bureau of the Census, *Current Population Reports*, P70-34. Washington, DC: U.S. Government Printing Office.

Eller, T. J. and Wallace Fraser. 1994. "Asset Ownership of Households: 1995." U.S. Bureau of the Census. *Current Population Reports,* P70-47. Washington, DC: U.S. Government Printing Office.

Englehardt, Gary V. and Christopher J. Mayer. 1994. "Gifts for Home Purchase and Housing Market Behavior." *New England Economic Review* (May/June): 47-58.

Families and Work Institute. 1995. *Women: The New Providers. A Study of Women's Views on Family, Work, Society and the Future.* Whirlpool Foundation Study, Part One. May.

Foster, Susan E. and Jack A. Brizius. 1993. "Caring Too Much? American Women and the Nation's Caregiving Crisis." Pp. 47-73 in *Women on the Front Lines.* Jessie Allen and Alan Pifer, eds. Washington, DC: Urban Institute Press.

Friedan, Betty. 1993. *The Fountain of Age.* New York: Simon and Shuster.

Friedman, Dana E. 1992. "The Corporate Commitment to Elder Care." New York: Families and Work Institute. January.

Gabor, Andrea. 1995. "Married with Househusband." *Working Woman* (November): 46, 48, 50, 96-98.

Genevay, Bonnie. 1993. "'Creating' Families: Older People Alone." Pp. 121-127 in *Families and Aging*, Linda Burton, ed. Amityville, NY: Baywood Publishing Company.

Genovese, Rosalie G. (ed.) 1984a. *Families and Change: Social Needs and Public Policies*. New York: Praeger.

Genovese, Rosalie G. 1984b. "The Role of Self-Help Networks in Meeting Family Needs." Pp. 321-333 in *Families and Change*, Rosalie G. Genovese, ed.

Glick, Paul C. and Sung-Ling Lin. 1986. "More Young Adults are Living with Their Parents: Who are They?" *Journal of Marriage and the Family* 48: 107-12.

Goldscheider, Frances K. and Calvin Goldscheider. 1988. "Family Structure and Conflict: Nest-Leaving Expectations of Young Adults and their Parents." *Journal of Marriage and the Family* 51: 87-97.

Goldscheider, F. and C. Goldscheider. 1993. "Whose Nest? A Two-Generational View of Leaving Home during the 1980s." *Journal of Marriage and the Family* 55 (4): 851-862.

Goldscheider, Frances K. and Celine LeBourdais. 1986. "The Decline in Age at Leaving Home, 1920-1979." *Sociology and Social Research* 70: 143-45.

Goldscheider, Frances K. and Calvin Goldscheider. 1994. "Leaving and Returning Home in 20th Century America." *Population Bulletin* 48, 4 (March).

Goldscheider, Frances K. and Julie DaVanzo. 1985. "Living Arrangements and the Transition to Adulthood." *Demography* 22: 545-63.

Goldscheider, Frances K. and Linda J. Waite. 1987. "Nest-leaving Patterns and the Transition to Marriage for Young Men and Women." *Journal of Marriage and the Family* 49: 507-516.

Goldscheider, Frances K. and Linda J. Waite. 1991. *New Families, No Families? The Transformation of the American Home*. Berkeley, CA: University of California Press.

Greenberg, Polly. 1985. "The Empty Nest Syndrome." Pp. 278-286 in *Marriage and Family: Coping with Change*, Leonard Cargan, ed. Belmont CA: Wadsworth.

Grigsby, Jill and Jill B. McGowan. 1986. "Still in the Nest: Adult Children Living with Their Parents." *Sociology and Social Research* 70: 146-148.

Hagestad, Gunhild O. 1988. "Demographic Change and Life Course: Some Emerging Trends in the Family Realm." *Family Relations* 37: 405-410.

Harel, Zev, Edward A. McKinney, and Michael Willams (eds.). 1990. *Black Aged: Understanding Diversity and Service Needs*. Newbury Park, CA: Sage Publications.

Harrington, Walt. 1995. "Falling Out of the Middle Class." *Washington Post Magazine*. April 23: 11-17, 24-27.

Hartmann, Heidi. 1995. "The Recent Past and Near Future for Women Workers: Addressing Remaining Barriers." Presented at the 75th Anniversary Conference, Women's Bureau, Washington, DC "Working Women Count: Yesterday, Today, and Tomorrow," May 20.

Hayward, Mark D. and Mei-Chun Liu. 1992. "Men and Women in their Retirement Years: A Demographic Profile." Pp. 23-50 in *Families and Retirement*, Maximiliane Szinovacz, David J. Ekerdt, and Barbara H. Vinick, eds. Newbury Park, CA: Sage Publications.

Himes, C. L. 1992. "Future Caregivers: Projected Family Structures of Older Persons." *Journal of Gerontology* 47(1): S17-S26.

Hirshorn, B. A. 1991. "Sharing or Competition: Multiple Views of the Intergenerational Flow of Society's Resources." *Marriage and Family Review* 16: 175-193.

Hofferth, Sandra L. 1984. "Kin Networks, Race and Family Structure." *Journal of Marriage and the Family* 46: 791-806.

Hogan, Dennis P. et al. 1990. "Race, Kin Networks and Assistance to Mother-Headed Families." *Social Forces* 68: 797-812.

"Home Health Care." 1996. *Family Economics and Nutrition Review* 9(2): 34-36.

Hooyman, Nancy R. 1992. "Social Policy and Gender Inequities in Caregiving." Pp. 181-201 in *Gender, Families and Elder Care*, Jeffrey W. Dwyer and Raymond T. Coward, eds. Newbury Park, CA: Sage Publications.

Horowitz, Amy. 1985. "Sons and Daughters as Caregivers to Older Parents: Differences in Role Performance and Consequence." *The Gerontologist* 25: 612-617.

Hunter, Ski and Martin Sundel (eds.). 1989. *Midlife Myths: Issues, Findings and Practice*. Newbury Park, CA: Sage Publications.

Institute for Women's Policy Research (IWPR). 1995. "The Economic Impact of Contingent Work on Women and Families." *Research in Brief*. Washington, DC: IWPR, September.

Jacobs, Ruth Harriet. 1993. "Expanding Social Roles for Older Women." Pp. 191-219 in *Women on the Front Lines* ed. Jessie Allen and Alan Pifer. Washington, DC: The Urban Institute Press.

Jendrek, M. P. 1994. "Grandparents Who Parent Their Grandchildren: Circumstances and Decisions." *The Gerontologist* 34(2): 206-216.

Jewell, K. Sue. 1988. "The Changing Character of Black Families: The Effects of Differential Social and Economic Gains." *Journal of Social and Behavioral Sciences* 33: 143-154.

Kain, Edward L. 1990. *The Myth of Family Decline: Understanding Families in a World of Rapid Change*. Lexington, MA: Lexington Books.

King, Miriam. 1988. *Changes in the Living Arrangements of the Elderly: 1960-2030*. Special Study, Congressional Budget Office. Washington, DC: Government Printing Office.

King, V. and G. H. Elder. 1995. "American Children View Their Grandparents: Linked Lives Across Three Rural Generations." *Journal of Marriage and the Family* 57(1): 165-177.

Kivett, Vera R. and R. Max Learner. 1982. "Situational Influences on the Morale of Older Rural Adults in Child-Shared Housing: A Comparative Analysis." *The Gerontologist* 22: 100-106.

Kornhaber, Arthur. 1996. *Contemporary Grandparenting*. Thousand Oaks, CA: Sage Publications.

Kornhaber, Arthur and Kenneth L. Woodward. 1991. *Grandparents, Grandchildren: The Vital Connection*. New Brunswick, NJ: Transaction [Rutgers].

Krout, John A. 1993. *Providing Community-based Services to the Rural Elderly*. Newbury Park, CA: Sage Publications.

Kulis, Stephen S. 1991. *Why Honor thy Father and Mother? Class, Mobility, and Family Ties in Later Life*. New York: Garland.

Kuriasky, Joan A. 1994. "Moving Toward Pension Equity." *Women and Pensions*. Washington, DC: OWL for the Women's Pension Policy Consortium.

Larson, Jan. 1996. "Temps Are Here to Stay." *American Demographics* 18, 2 (February): 26-31.

Lav, Iris J. and Edward B. Lazere. 1996. *A Hand Up: How State Earned Income Credits Help Families Escape Poverty*. Washington, DC: Center on Budget and Policy Priorities. January.

Lawlor, Julia. 1995. "Why Companies Should Care." *Working Woman* (June): 38-41.

Lawton, Leora, Merril Silverstein, and Vern Bengston. 1994. "Affection, Social Contact, and Geographic Distance Between Adult Children and Their Parents." *Journal of Marriage and the Family* 56 (February): 57-68.

Lee, G., J. Dwyer, and R. Coward. 1993. "Gender Differences in Parent Care: Demographic Factors and Same-Gender Preferences." *Journal of Gerontology: Social Sciences* 48: S9-S16.

Leonard, Frances. 1993a. *The Future of Housing: Old, Alone and Female in the 21st Century*. Washington, DC: Older Women's League.

Levinson, Daniel J. 1978. *The Seasons of a Man's Life*. New York: Ballantine Books.

Lin, Ge and Peter A. Rogerson. 1994. "Elderly Parents and the Geographic Availability of Their Adult Children." Department of Geography, State University of New York at Buffalo (December).

Littwin, Susan. 1986. *The Postponed Generation: Why American Youth are Growing Up Later*. New York: William Morrow.

Logan, John R. and Glenna Spitze. 1996. *Family Ties: Enduring Relations Between Parents and their Adult Children*. Philadelphia, PA: Temple University Press.

Loomis, Laura Spencer, and Alan Booth. 1995. "Multigenerational Caregiving and Well-Being: The Myth of the Beleaguered Sandwich Generation." *Journal of Family Issues* 16, 2(March): 131-148.

Lopata, Helena Z. 1995. *Current Widowhood: Myths and Realities*. Thousand Oaks, CA: Sage Publications.

Mahar, Maggie. 1992a. "Trading Places." *Working Woman* (July): 56-58, 61, 71.

Mahar, Maggie. 1992b. "No Bull Advice." *Working Woman* (October): 71-73, 96, 101.

Malveaux, Julianne. 1993. "Race, Poverty, and Women's Aging." Pp. 167-190 in *Women on the Front Lines,* Jessie Allen and Alan Pifer, eds. Washington, DC: The Urban Institute Press.

Mancini, Jay A. (ed.). 1992. "Intergenerational Relationships." *Journal of Family Issues* 13, 4(December): entire issue.

Markides, K. S., J. S. Boldt, and L. A. Ray. 1986. "Sources of Helping and Intergenerational Solidarity: A Three Generations Study of Mexican Americans." *Journal of Gerontology: Social Sciences* 42: 506-571.

Marks, Nadine F. 1993. *Caregiving Across the Lifespan: A New National Profile*. NSFH Working Paper No. 55. Madison, WI: Center for Demography and Ecology, University of Wisconsin.

Masnick, George S. and John R. Pitkin. 1983. "The Baby Boom and the Squeeze on Multigenerational Households." Working Paper #W83-6. Joint Center for Urban Studies of MIT and Harvard University, (July).

Masumura, Wilfred. 1995. "Dynamics of Economic Well-Being: Income, 1991 to 1992." *Current Population Reports*. Household Economic Studies P70-49. Washington, DC: U.S. Bureau of the Census (August).

Matthews, Sarah H. and Tena Tarler Rosner. 1988. "Shared Filial Responsibility: The Family as a Primary Caregiver." *Journal of Marriage and the Family* 50: 185-196.

McAdoo, Harriette Pipes. 1982. "Black Mothers and the Extended Family Support Network." Pp. 125-144 in *The Black Woman,* La Frances Rodgers-Rose, ed. Beverly Hills, CA: Sage Publications.

McLanahan, S. S. and A. B. Sorenson. 1985. "Life Events and Psychological Well-Being Over the Life Course." Pp. 217-238 in *Life Course Dynamics,* G. H. Elder, ed. Ithaca, NY: Cornell University Press.

McLanahan, S. S. and R. A. Monson. 1990. "Caring for the Elderly: Prevalence and Consequences." *NSFH Working Paper No. 18*. Center for Demography and Ecology, University of Wisconsin-Madison. December.

Menaghan, E. G. 1994. "The Daily Grind: Work Stressors, Family Patterns, and Intergenerational Outcomes." In *Stress and Mental Health: Contemporary Issues and Prospects for the Future,* William B. Avison and Ian Gotlib, eds. New York: Plenum Publishing Corp.

Minkler, Meredith and Kathleen M. Roe. 1992. *Grandmothers as Caregivers: Raising Children of the Crack Cocaine Epidemic*. Family Caregiver Applications Series, Volume 2 (Winter). Newbury Park, CA: Sage Publications.

Mitchell, Barbara A., Andrew V. Wister, and Thomas K. Burch. 1989. "The Family Environment and Leaving the Parental Home." *Journal of Marriage and the Family* 51: 605-613.

Moen, Phyllis, Donna Dempster McClain, and Robin M. Williams, Jr. 1989. "Social Integration and Longevity: An Event History Analysis of Women's Roles and Resilience." *American Sociological Review* 54, 4(August): 635-647.

Moen, P., J. Robison, and V. Fields. 1994. "Women's Work and Caregiving Roles: A Life Course Approach." *Journal of Gerontology: Social Sciences* 49: S176-S186.

Montgomery, R.J.V. and B. A. Hirshorn. 1991. "Current and Future Family Help with Long-Term Care Needs of the Elderly." *Research on Aging* 13: 171-204.

Morgan, Leslie A. 1992. "Marital Status and Retirement Plans: Do Widowhood and Divorce Make a Difference?" Pp. 114-126 in *Families and Retirement,* Maximiliane Scinovacz, David J. Ekerdt, and Barbara H. Vinick, eds. Newbury Park, CA: Sage Publications.

Morris, Betsy. 1996. "The Future of Retirement." *Fortune* (August 19): 86-94.

Mutran, Elizabeth. 1985. "Intergenerational Support among Blacks and Whites: Response to Culture or Socioeconomic Differences." *Journal of Gerontology* 40: 382-389.

National Commission for Employment Policy. 1995. *Unemployment Insurance: Barriers to Access for Women and Part-Time Workers*. Research Report No. 95-06. July. Washington, DC: National Commission for Employment Policy, U.S. Department of Labor.

Neal, Margaret B. et al. 1993. *Balancing Work and Caregiving for Children, Adults, and Elders*. Family Caregiver Applications Series, Vol. 3 (Winter). Newbury Park, CA: Sage Publications.

Nelson, Rob and Jon Cowan. 1994. *Revolution X: A Survival Guide for Our Generation*. New York: Penguin.

Norton, Arthur J. and Luisa F. Miller. 1992. "Marriage, Divorce, and Remarriage in the 1990's." *Current Population Reports Series P-23*, No. 180. U.S. Bureau of the Census, (December).

Older Women's League. 1993. "Room for Improvement: The Lack of Affordable, Adaptable and Accessible Housing for Midlife and Older Women." *1993 Mother's Day Report*.

Older Women's League. 1994. "Women and Pensions." Washington, DC: Older Women's League.

Older Women's League. 1995. "The Path to Poverty: An Analysis of Women's Retirement Income." Washington, DC: Older Women's League.

O'Rand, Angela M., John C. Henretta, and Margaret L. Krecker. 1992. "Family Pathways to Retirement." Pp. 81-98 in *Families and Retirement,* Maximiliane Scinovacz, David J. Ekerdt, and Barbara H. Vinick, eds. Newbury Park, CA: Sage Publications.

Peterson, Peter G. 1996. *Will America Grow Up Before It Grows Old? How the Coming Social Security Crisis Threatens You, Your Family, and Your Country.* New York: Random House.

Pett, Marjorie A., Nancy Lang, and Anita Gander. 1992. "Late-Life Divorce: Its Impact on Family Rituals." *Journal of Family Issues* (December): 526-552.

Pfeifer, Susan and Marvin B. Sussman. 1991. *Families: Intergenerational and Generational Connections.* Binghamton, NY: Haworth. Monograph published simultaneously as *Marriage and Family Review,* Vol. 16.

Pifer, Alan. "Meeting the Challenge: Implications for Policy and Practice." Pp. 241-252 in *Women on the Front Lines,* Jessie Allen and Alan Pifer, eds. Washington, DC: The Urban Institute Press.

Pillemer, Karl and K. McCartney (eds.). 1991. *Parent-Child Relations Across the Lifespan.* Hillsboro, NJ: Erlbaum.

Pillemer, Karl and J. Jill Suitor. 1991a. "Sharing a Residence with an Adult Child: A Cause of Psychological Distress in the Elderly?" *American Journal of Orthopsychiatry* 61,1(January): 144-148.

Pillemer, Karl and J. Jill Suitor. 1991b. "Will I Ever Escape My Child's Problems? Effects of Adult Children's Problems on Elderly Parents." *Journal of Marriage and the Family* 53, 3(August): 585-594.

Pogrebin, Letty Gottin. 1996. *Getting Over Getting Older: An Intimate Journey.* Boston: Little, Brown.

Popenoe, David. 1988. *Disturbing the Nest: Family, Change and Decline in Modern Societies.* New York: Aldine de Gruyter.

Presser, H. B. 1989. "Some Economic Complexities of Child Care Provided by Grandmothers." *Journal of Marriage and the Family* 51: 589-591.

Pruchno, Rachel. 1995. "Grandparents in American Society: Review of Recent Literature." Washington, DC: National Institute on Aging (September).

Riche, Martha Farnsworth. 1990. "Boomerang Age." *American Demographics* (May): 25-30, 52-53.

Riley, Matilda White. 1983. "The Family in an Aging Society: A Matrix of Latent Relationships." *Journal of Family Issues,* 4, 3(September): 439-454.

Rogerson, Peter A., Richard H. Weng, and Ge Lin. 1993. "The Spatial Separation of Parents and Their Adult Children." *Annals of the Association of American Geographers,* 83, 4(December): 656-671.

Room for Improvement: The Lack of Affordable, Adaptable, and Accessible Housing for Midlife and Older Women. 1993. Washington, DC: Older Women's League.

Rosenthal, Carolyn J. 1985. "Kinkeeping in the Familial Division of Labor." *Journal of Marriage and the Family* 47: 965-974.

Rossi, A. S. and P. H. Rossi. 1990. *Of Human Bonding: Parent-Child Relations across the Life Course*. Social Institutions and Social Change. New York: Aldine de Gruyter.

Ruggles, Steven and Ron Goeken. 1990. "Race and Multigenerational Family Structure, 1900 to 1980: Preliminary Findings." Paper presented at The Albany Conference on "Demographic Perspectives on the American Family: Patterns and Prospects," April 6.

Ryscavage, Paul. 1995. "Dynamics of Economic Well-Being: Labor Force, 1991 to 1993." *Current Population Reports*, Household Economic Studies, P70-48. August.

Saluter, Arlene. 1989. "Singleness in America." Pp. 1-12 in *Studies in Marriage and the Family*. Current Population Reports, Series P-23, No. 162. Washington, DC: U.S. Government Printing Office.

Sanders, G. F. and W. Trygstad. 1989. "Stepgrandparents and Grandparents: The View from Young Adults." *Family Relations* 38 (1): 71-74.

Schnaiberg, Allan and Sheldon Goldenberg. 1989. "From Empty Nest to Crowded Nest: The Dynamics of Incompletely-Launched Young Adults." *Social Problems* 36, 3: 251-269.

Seavey, Dorothy K. 1996. *Back to Basics: Women's Poverty and Welfare Reform*. Wellesley, MA: Center for Research on Women, Wellesley College.

Seccombe, Karen. 1992. "Employment, the Family and Employer-Based Policies." Pp. 165-180 in *Gender, Families and Elder Care,* Jeffrey W. Dwyer and Raymond T. Coward, eds. Newbury Park, CA: Sage Publications.

Shanas, Ethel. 1980. "Older People and their Families: The New Pioneers." *Journal of Marriage and the Family* 42: 9-15.

Sheehy, Gail. 1976. *Passages: Predictable Crises of Adult Life*. New York: Bantam.

Sheehy, Gail. 1995. "The Pursuit of Passion: Lessons From the World of Wisewomen." *Modern Maturity* (July-August): 42-46, 89.

Shehan, Constance L., Donna H. Berardo, and Felix M. Berardo. 1984. "The Empty Nest is Filling Again: Implications for Parent-Child Relations." *Parenting Studies* 1(2): 67-73.

Short, Kathleen and Martina Shea. 1995. "Beyond Poverty, Extended Measures of Well-Being: 1992." *Current Population Reports* Household Economic Studies. P70-50RV. Washington, DC: U.S. Bureau of the Census. November.

Siegel, J. S. 1993. *A Generation of Change: A Profile of America's Older Population*. New York: Russell Sage Foundation.

Skolnick, Arlene. 1991. *Embattled Paradise: The American Family in a Age of Uncertainty*. New York: Basic Books.

Smith, James P. 1995. "Unequal Wealth and Incentives to Save." *Documented Briefing*. Santa Monica, CA: RAND.

Smolowe, Jill. 1990. "To Grandmother's House We Go: More and more senior citizens are missing out on retirement while they serve as surrogate parents for their grandchildren." *Time* (November 5): 86-87.

Spalter-Roth, Roberta and Heidi I. Hartmann. 1988. *Unnecessary Losses: Costs to Americans of the Lack of Family and Medical Leave*. Washington, DC: Institute for Women's Policy Research.

Spitze, Glenna and John R. Logan. 1989. "Gender Differences in Family Support: Is There a Payoff?" *The Gerontologist* 29: 108-113.

Spitze, Glenna and John R. Logan. 1990. "Sons, Daughters, and Intergenerational Social Support." *Journal of Marriage and the Family* 52: 420-430.

Stein, Linda. 1995. "Love and Money: Live-in Couples Figure the Cost of Family Values." *Modern Maturity* (May-June): 44, 72, 73.

Steinmetz, Suzanne K. 1988. *Duty Bound: Elder Abuse and Family Care*. Newbury Park, CA: Sage Publications.

Steinmetz, Suzanne K. (ed.) 1988. *Family and Support Systems Across the Life Span*. New York: Plenum.

Stone, Robyn. 1989. "The Feminization of Poverty Among the Elderly." *Women's Studies Quarterly* 17 (Spring/Summer). Reprinted by the National Center for Health Services Research and Health Care Technology Assessment, U.S. Department of Health and Human Services.

Stone, R., G. L. Cafferata, and J. Sangl. 1987. "Caregivers of the Frail Elderly: A National Profile." *The Gerontologist* 27: 616-626.

Suitor, Jill and Karl Pillemer. 1987. "The Presence of Adult Children: A Source of Stress for Elderly Couples' Marriages?" *Journal of Marriage and the Family* 49: 717-725.

Suitor, Jill and Karl Pillemer. 1988. "Explaining Intergenerational Conflict When Adult Children and Elderly Parents Live Together." *Journal of Marriage and the Family* 50: 1037-47.

Suitor, Jill and Karl Pillemer. 1991. "Family Conflict When Adult Children and Elderly Parents Share a Home." Pp. 179-199 in *Parent-Child Relations Throughout Life*, K. Pillemer and K. M. Cartney, eds. Hillsdale, NJ: Lawerence Erlbaum.

Szinovacz, Maximiliane, David J. Ekerdt, and Barbara H. Vinick (eds.). 1992a. *Families and Retirement*. Newbury Park, CA: Sage Publications.

Szinovacz, Maximiliane, David J. Ekerdt, and Barbara H. Vinick. 1992b. "Families and Retirement: Avenues for Future Research." Pp. 236-261 in *Families and Retirement*, Maximiliane Szinovacz, David J. Ekerdt and Barbara H. Vinick, eds. Newbury Park, CA: Sage Publications.

Taeuber, Cynthia M. 1992. "Sixty-Five Plus in America." *Current Population Reports*, Special Studies P23-178RV. Washington, DC: U.S. Bureau of the Census.

Taeuber, Cynthia M. and Jessie Allen. 1993. "Women in Our Aging Society: The Demographic Outlook." Pp. 11-45 in *Women on the Front Lines,* Jessie Allen and Alan Pifer, eds. Washington, DC: The Urban Institute Press.

Taylor, Susan Champlin. 1993. "The End of Retirement." *Modern Maturity* (October-November 1993): 32-39.

Taylor, Susan Champlin. 1994. "What Child is This..." *Modern Maturity* (December 1993-January 1994): 42-47, 77.

Treas, Judith. 1995. "Older Americans in the 1990s and Beyond." *Population Bulletin* 50, 2(May).

Troll, Lillian. 1989. "Myths of Midlife Intergenerational Relationships." Pp. 210-231 in *Midlife Myths: Issues, Findings and Practices,* Ski Hunter and Martin Sundel, eds. Newbury Park, CA: Sage Publications.

U.S. Bureau of the Census. 1987. "Marital Status and Living Arrangements: March 1986." *Current Population Reports*, Series P-20, No. 410. Washington, DC: U.S. Government Printing Office.

U.S. Bureau of the Census. 1988. "Who's Helping Out? Support Networks Among American Families." *Current Population Reports*, Series P-70, No. 13. Washington, DC: U.S. Government Printing Office.

U.S. Bureau of the Census. 1992. "Workers with Low Earnings: 1964 to 1990." *Current Population Reports*, Series P-60, No. 178. Washington, DC: U.S. Government Printing Office.

U.S. General Accounting Office. 1992. *The Changing Workforce: A Comparison of Federal and Nonfederal Work/Family Programs and Approaches.* Report to Congressional Committees (April).

U.S. Merit Systems Protection Board. 1992. *A Question of Equity: Women and the Glass Ceiling in the Federal Government.* A Report to the President and Congress of the United States (October).

Walker, Alexis J. and Clara C. Pratt. 1991a. "Daughters Help to Elderly Mothers." *Journal of Marriage and the Family* 53, 1(February): 13-27.

Walker, Alexis J. and Clara C. Pratt. 1991b. "Daughters' Help to Mothers: Intergenerational Aid Versus Caregiving." *Journal of Marriage and the Family* 53(1): 3-12.

Walker, Alexis J. and Clara C. Pratt. 1995. "Informal Caregiving to Aging Family Members: A Critical Review." *Family Relations* 4, 4(October): 402-411.

Walker, Alexis J. and L. Thompson. 1983. "Intimacy and Intergenerational Aid and Contact among Mothers and Daughters." *Journal of Marriage and the Family* 45(4): 841-849.

Walker, Paul L. 1991. "Eldercare: As the Baby Boomers become the sandwich generation, aging moves to the front of American concerns." *Employee Assistance* (April): 32-36.

Ward, Russell A. and Glenna Spitze. 1992. "Consequences of Parent-Adult Child Coresidence." *Journal of Family Issues* 13, 1(December): 553-572.

Ward, R., J. Logan and G. Spitze. 1992. "The Influence of Parents and Child Needs on Coresidence in Middle and Later Life." *Journal of Marriage and the Family* 54: 209-221.

Wellman, B. and N. S. Wortley. 1990. "Brothers' Keepers: Situating Kinship Relations in Broader Networks of Social Support." In *Aiding and Aging: The Coming Crisis in Support for the Elderly by Kin and State*, J. Mogey, ed. Contributions to Aging, No. 17. Westport, CT: Greenwood Press.

Whitbeck, L., D. R. Hoyt, and S. M. Huck. 1994. "Early Family Relationships, Intergenerational Solidarity, and Support Provided to Parents by Their Adult Children." *Journal of Gerontology: Social Sciences.* 49(2): S85-S94.

White, Lynn and John N. Edwards. 1990. "Emptying the Nest and Parental Well-Being: An Analysis of National Panel Data." *American Sociological Review* 55(April): 235-242.

White-Means, Shelley I. and Michael C. Thornton. 1990. "Ethnic Differences in the Production of Informal Home Health Care." *The Gerontologist* 30 (December): 758-768.

Wilson, William Julius. 1996. *When Work Disappears: The World of the New Urban Poor*. New York: Alfred A. Knopf.

Winik, Lyric Wallwork. 1995. "How Much Can I Give?" *Parade Magazine.* (January 29).

Women's Bureau. 1993. *Midlife Women Speak Out: Assessing Job Training* and *The Status of Working Women: A Statistical Profile of Midlife Women Aged 35-54*. Washington, DC: Women's Bureau, Office of the Secretary, U.S. Department of Labor (October).

Worobey, J. L. and R. J. Angel. 1990. "Poverty and Health: Older Minority Women and Rise of the Female-Headed Household." *Journal of Health and Social Behavior*, 31(4): 370-383.

Zal, H. Michael. 1992. *The Sandwich Generation: Caught Between Growing Children and Aging Parents*. New York: Plenum.

Zill, Nicholas and Christine Winquist Nord. 1994. *Running in Place: How American Families are Faring in a Changing Economy and an Individualistic Society*. Washington, DC: Child Trends, Inc.

NEWSPAPER ARTICLES

"A Bigger Family Stays Closer to the Nest." 1994. *Wall Street Journal* (April 11): B1.

Ansberry, Clare. 1990. "The Rising Prosperity of America's Retirees is Unevenly Spread." *Wall Street Journal* (November 13): A1, A16.

Arden-Smith, Tara. 1996. "U.S. Acts to Expand 'Reverse Mortgage' Option for Elderly." *Wall Street Journal* (July 19): B6.

Asinof, Lynn. 1993. "The Talk You Must Have With Your Parents." *Wall Street Journal* (March 26): C1.

Barringer, Felicity. 1991. "Changes in U.S. Households: Single Parents Amid Solitude." *New York Times* (June 7): 18.

Bernard, Joan Kelly. 1994. "Remote Chance for Romance: It's Hard for Young Adults to Make the Moves When They Haven't Moved from Home." *Rochester Democrat and Chronicle* (December 29). Reprinted from *Newsday*.

Blumenthal, Robin Goldwyn. 1996. "Midlife Brooding: Some Parents Find Third Time a Charm." *Wall Street Journal* (March 29): A1, A4.

Chase, Marilyn. 1995. "Pick a Nursing Home for the Best of an Elder's Abilities." *Wall Street Journal* (April 17): B1.

Clements, Jonathan. 1995a. "Dear Mom and Dad: Here's Something That's Easier to Read Than Discuss." *Wall Street Journal* (April 11): C1.

Clements, Jonathan. 1995b. "Delaying Social Security Benefits May Not Be As Smart As You Think." *Wall Street Journal* (April 18): C-1.

Cowan, Alison L. 1989. "Parenthood II: The Nest Won't Stay Empty." *New York Times* (March 12): 1.

Duff, Christina. 1994. "Cool Pad, Fab Food, One Catch: Mom Lives There Too." *Wall Street Journal* (September 12): A1, A8.

Duff, Christina. 1996. "Passing the Bucks: Aging Boomers Cut the Cord But Can't Let Go of the Wallet." *Wall Street Journal* (July 8): A1, A4.

Egan, T. 1992. "When Children Can't Afford Parents." *New York Times* (March 29): E7.

Finder, Alan. 1990. "Apartment Doubling-Up Rising in Working Class." *New York Times* (September 25): A1, B6.

Gabriel, Trip. 1996. "Holiday Travelers Make Room for Grandma." *New York Times* (July 14): 1, 20.

Garner, Jack. 1996. "Half Full, Half Empty." *Rochester Democrat and Chronicle* (August 29): 1C, 2C.

Graham, Ellen. 1995. "Their Careers: Count on Nothing and Work Like a Demon." First in a series, "The Baby Boom Hits 50." *Wall Street Journal* (October 31): B1, B10.

Graham, Ellen. 1996. "Craving Closer Ties, Strangers Come Together as Family." *Wall Street Journal* (March 4): B1, B5.

Gross, Jane. 1991a. "Help for Grandparents Caught Up in Drug War." *New York Times* (April 14): 18.

Gross, Jane. 1991b. "More Young Single Men Hang Onto Apron Strings." *New York Times* (June 16): 1, 18.

Herndon, Lucia. 1996. "Home Again." *Rochester Democrat and Chronicle* (August 15): 3C.

"How Families Will Cope With An Aging Population." 1992. *USA Today* (April 9): 11A.

Jeffrey, Nancy Ann. 1995. "Timely Financial Plan Softens Blow of Divorce." *Wall Street Journal* (April 21): C1.

Johnston, David Cay. 1995. "Who's Been Eating My Nest Egg: How Some Bosses are Raiding 401(k)'s." *Wall Street Journal* (November 26): 1, 6.

Kristof, Nicholas D. 1996. "Aging World, New Wrinkles." *New York Times* (September 22): E1, E5.

Kuttner, Lawrence. 1988. "Parent and Child: When Young Adults Head Back Home, Set a Time Limit and Don't Panic." *New York Times* (July 14).

Lipovenko, Dorothy. 1996. "Death of Children Price of Long Life." *Toronto Globe and Mail* (March 28): A1, A6.

Lowenstein, Roger. 1995. "Will Flat Wages Beget Future Trouble?" *Wall Street Journal* (October 23): C1.

Lowenstein, Roger. 1996. "The Fixes Social Security Doesn't Need." *Wall Street Journal* (April 11): C1.

Malcolm, Andrew H. 1991. "Helping Grandparents Who Are Parents Again." *New York Times* (November 19).

Martin, Douglas. 1991. "Now the Work That's Never Done Is Grandmother's." *New York Times* (May 12): E6.

"More Young Adults are Living with Their Parents." 1994. *Rochester Democrat and Chronicle* (June 19).

Morrison, Mark. 1996. "One Vacation, Three Generations." *USA Weekend* (October 11-13): 14.

Noble, Barbara Presley. 1994. "Old Age is No Place for Sissies." *New York Times* (February 6): F29.

O'Connell, Vanessa. 1996. "Boosting Your Earnings in an Uncertain World." *Wall Street Journal* (February 9): C1, C16.

Otten, Alan L. 1990. "Grown Kids at Home: Most Parents Don't Mind." *Wall Street Journal* (September 26): B-1.

Otten, Alan L. 1991. "Parental Nest Still Gives Aid to Young Adults." *Wall Street Journal* (January 14): B-1.

Otten, Alan L. 1994. "Grandparenting Becomes a Full-Time Pursuit." *Wall Street Journal* (March 7): B1.

Pollock, Ellen Joan. 1996. "Ambition Imbalance: She Wants to Work, He Wants to Golf." *Wall Street Journal* (April 11): A1, A12.

Powers, Helen. 1996. "A Widow's Walk on the Wild Side." *New York Times* (April 28): F11.

"Roles in the Home Can Vary Over Time." 1990. *Wall Street Journal* (August 3): B-1.

Romero, Dennis. 1994. "Social Security: Payoffs Pit Young vs. 'Golf-Cart Grannies.'" *Sarasota Herald Tribune* (December 28).

Rosen, Ellen. 1996a. "A Couple in the Middle." *Rochester Democrat and Chronicle* (July 14): 1C, 4C.

Rosen, Ellen. 1996b. "In Grandmother's House." *Rochester Democrat and Chronicle* (August 22): 1C, 6C.

Rosewicz, Barbara. 1996. "Here Comes the Bride...and for the Umpteenth Time." *Wall Street Journal* (September 10): B1, B14.

Rowland, Mary. 1991. "The Awkward Full Nest Syndrome." *New York Times* (February 24): F16.

Schultz, Ellen E. 1994. "Survivors Find New Help With Financial Decisions." *Wall Street Journal* (September 16): C1.

Schultz, Ellen E. 1995. "Frittered Away: Offered a Lump Sum, Many Retirees Blow It and Risk Their Future." *Wall Street Journal* (July 31): A1, A6.

Schultz, Ellen E. 1996a. "Some Workers Find Retirement Nest Eggs Full of Strange Assets." *Wall Street Journal* (June 5): A1, A8.

Schultz, Ellen E. 1996b. "Color Tile's 401(k) Plan Runs Aground." *Wall Street Journal* (June 8): C1, C29.

Scott, Sophfronia. 1991. "What Do We Do Now? Facing a Dismal Job Market, the Class of '91 Tries Interview Rehearsals, Internships, Even--yikes!--Living at Home." *Time* (May 20): 46.

Shellenbarger, Sue. 1992. "Employees Are Reticent About Caring for Elders." *Wall Street Journal* (Nov. 11): B1.

Shellenbarger, Sue. 1993. "Firms Try Harder, But Often Fail, to Help Workers Cope with Elder-Care Problems." *Wall Street Journal* (June 23): B1, B6.

Shellenbarger, Sue. 1994a. "More Day Care Centers Help the Aging Attend to the Aged." *Wall Street Journal* (March 17): B1.

Shellenbarger, Sue. 1994b. "Elderly Relatives Part of Relocation Deals." *Wall Street Journal* (May 11): B1.

Shellenbarger, Sue. 1995a. "A Worker's Guide to Finding Help in Caring for an Elder." *Wall Street Journal* (April 5): B1.

Shellenbarger, Sue. 1995b. "In Caring for Elders, Sometimes Less Can Accomplish More." *Wall Street Journal* (August 2): B1.

Shellenbarger, Sue. 1996. "Care-giver Duties Make Generation Xers Anything But Slackers." *Wall Street Journal* (May 22): B1.

Stecklow, Steve. 1996. "Trustee for New Era is Suing Prudential." *Wall Street Journal* (June 27): A3.

"Study of Transamerica Workers Shows High Costs of Elder Care." 1988. *Investors Daily* (April 20): 25.

Toner, Robin. 1995. "No Free Rides: Generational Push Has Not Come to Shove." *New York Times* (December 31): E1, E4.

Uchitelle, Louis. 1995. "Retirement's Worried Face: For Many the Crisis is Now." *New York Times* (July 30): F1, F4, F5.

Uchitelle, Louis. 1996. "Not Making It: We're Leaner, Meaner and Going Nowhere Faster." *New York Times* (May 12): 1E, 4E.

Zladivar, R. A. 1995. "When It Works, EITC 'Much Better' than Welfare." *Rochester Democrat and Chronicle* (March 26).

"HOW-TO" ADVICE: BOOKS, ARTICLES AND GUIDES

Abramson, Betsy. 1991. *Mastering the Medicare Maze: An Essential Guide to Benefits, Appeals and Medicare.* Madison, WI: Center for Public Representation.

Adams, Jane. 1994. *I'm Still Your Mother: How to Get Along With Your Grown-Up Children for the Rest of Your Life.* New York: Dell.

Aging Parents and Common Sense: A Practical Guide for You and Your Parents. 1995. Sponsored by The Equitable Foundation and Children of Aging Parents (CAPS).

Alberts, Nuna. 1995. "Your Aging Parents: How to Help." *American Health* (April): 54-57, 92-95.

American Association of Retired Persons (AARP). 1988. *A Primer on Financial Management for Midlife and Older Women.* Washington: Consumer Affairs Section, AARP.

American Association of Retired Persons. 1989. *A Handbook About Care in the Home: Information on Home Health Services.* Washington, DC: Health Advocacy Services Program, AARP.

American Association of Retired Persons. 1991b. *Focus Your Future: A Woman's Guide to Retirement Planning.* Washington, DC: AARP.

American Association of Retired Persons. 1992c. *Returning to the Job Market: A Woman's Guide to Employment Planning.* Washington, DC: AARP.

American Association of Retired Persons. 1992d. *Tomorrow's Choices: Preparing Now for Future Legal, Financial, and Health Care Decisions.* Washington, DC: AARP.

American Association of Retired Persons. 1992e. *A Woman's Guide to Pension Rights.* Washington, DC: AARP.

American Association of Retired Persons. 1994b. "A Path for Caregivers." Washington, DC: AARP.

American Association of Retired Persons. 1994c. "'We Can Understand How You Feel': Tapping into the Benefits of Self-Help/Mutual Aid Groups." Washington, DC: AARP.

American Institute for Economic Research. 1995. "How to Avoid Financial Tangles." *Economic Education Bulletin* 35, 1 (January).

Bass, Deborah. 1990. *Caring Families: Supports and Interventions.* Silver Spring, MD: National Association of Social Workers.

Beardstown Ladies Investment Club, with Leslie Whitaker. 1994. *Common-Sense Investment Guide: How We Beat the Stock Market--and How You Can, Too.* New York: Hyperion.

Broussard, Cheryl D. 1995. *The Black Woman's Guide to Financial Independence: Smart Ways to Take Charge of Your Money, Build Wealth, and Achieve Financial Security.* New York: Penguin Books.

Carlin, V. F. 1987. *Where Can Mom Live? A Family Guide to Living Arrangements for Elderly Parents.* Lexington, MA: Lexington Books.

Carlin, V. F. and Ruth Mansberg. 1989. *If I Live to be 100. A Creative Housing Solution for Older People*. Princeton, NJ: Princeton Book Co.

Carpenter, Liz. 1994b. *Unplanned Parenthood*. New York: Random House.

Carter, Rosalynn and Susan K. Golant. 1994. *Helping Yourself Help Others: A Book for Caregivers*. New York: Time Books.

Chambers, Nancy. 1995. "Where to Turn for Help." *Working Woman* (June): 49.

Children of Aging Parents. 1990. "Nursing Home Evaluation Form."

Children of Aging Parents. 1992. "Adult Day Care." *The Capsule* 8, 1.

Children of Aging Parents. 1993. "Starting a Support Group for Caregivers of the Elderly." (Manual.)

Children of Aging Parents. n.d. "Tips for Caregivers," Volumes 1 and 2.

Cohen, Charles E. 1994. "Six Steps to a First-Class Retirement." *Working Woman*. (Sept.): 56-61.

De Yoe, Elizabeth. 1995. "How to Create a Financial Safety Net." *Working Woman* (September): 26, 27, 76, 79, 82.

Dolan, J. Michael. 1992. *How to Care for Your Aging Parents...and Still Have a Life of Your Own*. Los Angeles, CA.: Mulholland Pacific Press.

"Encouraging Women to Build Bigger Nest Eggs." 1994. *Working Age*. Special Issue on Older Women and the Changing Work Force, 10, 4(November/December): 2-4.

Estess, Patricia Schiff. 1994. "When Kids Don't Leave; How to Cope with Our Stay-At-Home Offspring." *Modern Maturity* (November-December): 56, 58, 90.

Family Service America. 1990. *The Family Guide to Elder Care: Making the Right Choices*. Milwaukee, WI: Family Service America.

Ferguson, Karen and Kate Blackwell. 1995. *Pensions in Crisis: Why the System is Failing America and How You Can Protect Your Future*. New York: Arcade Publishing.

Freudlich, Deborah. 1995. *Retirement Living Communities: A National Directory*. New York: Macmillan.

Galinsky, Ellen, James T. Bond, and Dana E. Friedman. 1993. *The Changing Workforce: Highlights from the National Study*. New York: Families and Work Institute.

Gibson, D. and R. Gibson. 1991. *The Sandwich Years: When Your Kids Need Friends and Your Parents Need Parenting*. Grand Rapids, MI: Baker Book House.

Giese, William. 1995. "Retirement: How Boomers Can Avoid a Bust." *Kiplinger's Personal Finance Magazine* (October): 51-57.

Greenberg, Vivian. 1989. *Your Best is Good Enough*. Lexington, MA: Lexington Books.

Greenberg, Vivian. 1996. "Setting Parameters." *The Sandwich Generation* (Spring): 4-5.

Hayes, Christopher L. and Jane M. Deren (eds.). 1990. *Pre-Retirement Planning for Women: Program Design and Research*. New York: Springer Publishing Company.

Heath, Angela. 1993. *Long Distance Caregiving: A Survival Guide for Far Away Caregivers*. San Luis Obispo, CA: Impact Publishers, American Source Books.

Hannon, Kerry. 1995. "Why the Rules are Different for Women." *Working Woman* (September): 20-22, 24, 78.

Hannon, Kerry. 1996. "Cyberhelp for Your Investment Portfolio." *Working Woman* (June): 23-24.

Horne, Jo. 1985. *Caregiving: Helping an Aging Loved One*. Glenview, IL: Scott, Foresman and Company.

Internal Revenue Service (IRS*). Pension and Annuity Income (Including Simplified General Rule)*. Publication 575.

Internal Revenue Service (IRS). *Looking Out for #2: A Married Couple's Guide to Understanding Your Benefit Choices at Retirement From a Defined Contribution Plan*. Publication 1565.

Internal Revenue Service (IRS). *Looking Out for #2: A Married Couple's Guide to Understanding Your Benefit Choices at Retirement From a Defined Benefit Plan*. Publication 1566.

Kaufman, Laura. 1996. "Women and Money: Taking Control and Making a Plan." *Women's Philanthropy* 4, 1(June): 1, 3-5.

Klingelhofer, Edwin. 1989. *Coping with Your Grown Children*. New York: Dell.

Kobliner, Beth. 1996. *Get a Financial Life: Personal Finance in Your Twenties and Thirties*. New York: Fireside.

Kuhn, Susan E. 1996a. "Creating a High-Powered 401(k) Strategy." *Fortune* (August 19): 133-134.

Kuhn, Susan E. 1996b. "Will a Bear Market Wreck Your Retirement Plans?" *Fortune* (August 19): 137-140.

Kupferberg, Audrey E. 1991. "Why We Moved Back: Can the Children Really Come Home Again?" *Parade Magazine* (December 22): 16-18.

Leonard, Frances. 1993b. *Money and the Mature Woman: The Independent Woman's Guide to Financial Security for Life*. Reading, MA: Addison-Wesley Publishing.

Levin, Nora Jean. 1993. *How to Care for Your Parents: A Handbook for Adult Children*. 3rd Ed. Friday Harbor, WA: Storm King Press.

Levine, David. 1995. "Your Aging Parents: Choosing a Nursing Home." *American Health* (June): 82-85.

Levitin, Nancy. 1994. *Retirement Rights: The Benefits of Growing Older*. New York: Avon Books.

Levy, Michael T. 1991. *Parenting Mom and Dad: A Guide for the Grown-Up Children of Aging Parents*. New York: Prentice-Hall.

Lindeman, Leslie. 1993. "Bootstrap Investing: Scared of Stocks? Try the Club Scene." *Modern Maturity* (October-November): 42-44, 82-83.

Longo, Tracey. 1995a. "Divvying Up Your Retirement Money." *Kiplinger's Personal Finance Magazine*. (August): 95-96.

Longo, Tracey. 1995b. "When Distant Parents Need Your Help." *Kiplinger's Personal Finance Magazine*. (December): 91-96.

Longo, Tracey. 1996. "How Singles Should Plan Their Finances." *Kiplinger's Personal Finance Magazine.* (May): 81-83.

Lynch, Peter, with John Rothschild. 1989. *One Up On Wall Street: How to Use What You Already Know to Make Money in the Market.* New York: Simon and Schuster.

Mall, E. Jane. 1990. *Caregiving: How to Care for Your Elderly Mother and Stay Sane.* New York: Ballantine.

McGurn, Sheelagh. 1992. *Under One Roof: Caring for an Aging Parent.* Park Ridge, IL: Parkside Publishing.

McLean, Bethany. 1996. "How Your 401(k) Stacks Up." *Fortune* (August 19): 124-130.

Mental Health Directory. 1990. Washington, DC: National Institute of Mental Health.

Moreau, Dan. 1996. "What to Do if the Ax Falls." *Kiplinger's Personal Finance Magazine,* (February): 91-94.

Morris, Betsy. 1996. "The Future of Retirement: It's Not What You Think." *Fortune* (August 19): 86-94.

Moss, Anne E. 1995. *Your Pension Rights at Divorce: What Women Need to Know.* Pension Rights Center, 918 16th St. NW, Suite 701, Washington, DC 20006.

"Multiple Marriages: How to Avoid Financial Traps." 1996. *The Sandwich Generation* (Spring): 14-15, 17.

National Center for Women and Retirement Research. 1990. *Social and Emotional Issues for Midlife Women.* Southampton, NY: National Center for Women and Retirement Research, Long Island University.

National Center for Women and Retirement Research. 1995a. *Long-Term Care for Women: How Will We Receive and Give Care.* Southampton, NY: National Center for Women and Retirement Research, Long Island University.

National Center for Women and Retirement Research. 1995b. *Looking Ahead to Your Financial Future.* Southampton, NY: National Center for Women and Retirement Research, Long Island University.

National Consumers League (NCL). 1995. *Consumer Tip: A Consumer's Guide to Life-Care Communities.* Available from NCL, 815 15th St. NW, #928-N, Washington, DC 20605.

National Directory of Retirement Facilities, 3rd Ed. 1991. Phoenix, AZ: Orynx Press.

National Institute on Adult Daycare. 1995. "Your Guide to Selecting an Adult Day Care Center." Washington, DC: National Council on the Aging, Inc.

National Institute of Mental Health. "If You're Over 65 and Feeling Depressed." (Call 1-800-421-4211).

"Navigating the Internet: A Compass for Individual Investors." 1996. *Individual Investor* 10, 3(June/July): 1-3.

New York State Journal for Elder Planning and Care. East Cottage Associates, 120 DeFreest Drive, Troy, NY 12180.

Norris, Jane. 1988. *Daughters of the Elderly: Building Partnerships in Caregiving*. Bloomington, IN: Indiana University Press.

"Nursing Homes: When a Loved One Needs Care." 1995. *Consumer Reports*. (August): 518-529.

"Nursing Home Contracts: What You Need to Know About Those Illegal Clauses." 1996. *The Sandwich Generation* (Spring): 21-24.

Okimoto, Jean Davies and Phyllis Jackson Stegall. 1987. *Boomerang Kids: How to Live with Adult Children Who Return Home*. Boston, MA: Little, Brown.

Oregon State University Extension Service. "Depression in Later Life: Recognition and Treatment." Available from OSU, #PNW347, Publication Orders, Dept. P, Agriculture Communications, Administrative Services, Room A422, Corvallis, OR 97331.

Patterson, Martha Priddy. 1993. *The Working Woman's Guide to Retirement: Saving and Investing Now for a Secure Future*. Englewood Cliffs, NJ: Prentice-Hall.

Polniaszek, Susan. 1991. *Long-Term Care: A Dollar and Sense Guide*. Washington, DC: United Seniors Health Cooperative. Available from the Cooperative, 1334 G Street, Suite 500, Washington, DC 20005.

Quinn, Jane Bryant. 1991. *Making the Most of Your Money*. New York: Simon and Schuster.

Razzi, Elizabeth. 1996. "Finding the Right Caregiver." *Kiplinger's Personal Finance Magazine*. (May): 67-68, 71, 73.

"Retirement Spending: Making Sure Your Money Will Last." 1995. *The Individual Investor* 9, 3(June/July): 1-3.

Rothchild, John. 1996. "How to Choose Your Advisors." *Fortune* (August 19): 171-176.

The Sandwich Generation. One year subscription is $14.00. Available from The Sandwich Generation, Box 132, Wickantunk, NJ 07765.

Savage, Terry. 1993. *New Money Strategies for the 1990s*. New York: HarperBusiness.

Schoenfeld, Eric. 1996. "Do It Yourself: How to Build Wealth with Individual Stocks." *Fortune* (August 19): 164-168.

Shane, Dorlene V. and United Seniors Health Center. 1991. *Finances After 50: Financial Planning for the Rest of Your Life*. New York: Harper and Row.

Shapiro, Barbara A. 1991. *The Big Squeeze: Balancing the Needs of Aging Parents, Dependent Children and YOU*. Bedford, MA: Mills and Sanderson.

Shapiro, Pat. 1994. "My House is Your House: Advance Planning Can Ease the Way When Parents Move in with Adult Kids." *AARP Bulletin* (November): 2.

Shelley, Florence D. 1988. *When Your Parents Grow Old.* New York: Harper and Row.

"Should I Quit My Job??? And Stay Home and Care for Mom?" 1996. *The Sandwich Generation* (Fall): 3-4.

Smith, Kerri S. 1992. *Caring for Your Aging Parents: A Sourcebook of Timesaving Techniques and Tips.* Lakewood, CO: American Source Books.

Smith, Shauna L. 1991. *Making Peace with Your Adult Children.* New York: Plenum Press.

Social Security Administration. 1995a. "Understanding Social Security." SSA Publication No. 05-10024 (January) (updated regularly).

Social Security Administration. 1995b. "When You Get Social Security Retirement or Survivors Benefits: What You Need to Know." SSA Publication No. 05-10077 (updated regularly).

Spraggins, Ellyn. 1995. "The Best Strategies for Your 401(k)." *Working Woman* (November): 36-40.

Sprinkle, Patricia H. 1996. *Women Home Alone: Learning to Thrive.* Grand Rapids, MI: Zondervan.

Standard and Poor's Stock Reports. Available from Standard and Poors, 25 Broadway, New York, NY 10004.

U.S. Department of Health and Human Services, Health Care Financing Administration. 1994. *Guide to Choosing a Nursing Home.* Baltimore, MD: U.S. Department of Health and Human Services.

U.S. Department of Health and Human Services, Health Care Financing Administration. 1995. *Your Medicare Handbook.* Publication No. HCFA 10050.

U.S. Department of Labor, Bureau of Labor Statistics. 1991. "Getting Back to Work." Washington, DC: U.S. Government Printing Office.

Value Line Investment Survey. Subscription available from Value Line, 220 E. 42nd St., New York, NY 10017.

Warren, Larkin. 1995. "Survival Lessons." *Working Woman* (June): 47-48, 74-75.

Werner, Anne and James Firman. 1994. *Home Care for Older People: A Consumer's Guide.* Washington, DC: United Seniors Health Cooperative. Available from the Cooperative, 1334 G Street, Suite 500, Washington, DC 20005.

White, Jerry and Mary White. 1991. *When Your Kids Aren't Kids Anymore.* Colorado Springs, CO: NavPress.

White, Shelby. 1995. *What Every Woman Should Know About Her Husband's Money.* New York: Random House.

"Who Pays for Nursing Homes?" 1995. *Consumer Reports* (September): 591-597. Reprints are available from CU/Reprints, 101 Truman Ave., Yonkers, NY 10703.

Wilcox, Melynda Dovel. 1996. "Not a Place to Sit and Watch the Traffic." *Kiplinger's Personal Finance Magazine* (June): 62-69.

Willis, Clint. 1995. "When to Talk About Money." *Working Woman* (June): 42-
    45, 72-73, 76.
Willis, Clint. 1996a. "Smart Investment Moves for Every Stage of Your Life."
    Working Woman (September): 29-40, 87.
Willis, Clint. 1996b. "The Five Most Expensive Mistakes Women Make."
    Working Woman (September): 42-46, 83.
Wyatt, John. 1996. "What You'll Need to Survive...and Prosper." *Fortune*
    (August 19): 99-106.
"Your Complete Guide to Financial Security." 1995. *Working Woman*
    (September): entire issue.

Author Index

Subject Index

About the Author

ROSALIE G. GENOVESE is a Visiting Scholar at the University of Rochester's Susan B. Anthony University Center. She is the editor of *Families and Change: Social Needs and Public Policies* and has written many articles, chapters and reports on public policy issues, urban and community planning, dual-career couples, and economic security for low-income women. In addition to program development and policy analysis for not-for-profit organizations in New York, Boston and Rochester, her experience includes teaching positions at the University of Massachusetts at Boston and colleges in the Rochester area. She also worked as a financial advisor for a prominent brokerage house.